FORMULATION AND ... DRUG

ACKNOWLEDGEMENTS

I deem it a pleasure and privilege to work under the joint supervision of **Dr. Amalesh Samanta,** Professor, Division of Microbiology, Dept. of Pharm. Tech., Jadavpur University and **Dr. Pintu Kumar De**, Principal & Professor, Dr. B. C. Roy College of Pharmacy and A.H.S., Durgapur. I express my deep gratitude and regards to my guides for their thoughtful and rational, propelling inspiration, informative and critical discussions, valuable suggestions and persistent encouragement throughout this research.

I am also extremely grateful to the **Vice Chancellor, Registrar & Dean** of the Faculty of Engineering and Technology, **Head, Department of Pharmaceutical Technology** of Jadavpur University and **Managing Director, Dr. B. C. Roy College of Pharmacy & AHS**, Durgapur for providing the facilities needed for my research work.

I acknowledge with gratitude the help and support I received from **Dr. Asish Kumar Mukhopadhyay**, Scientist E and his research fellow **Ronita De**, Division of Bacteriology, **National Institute of Cholera and Enteric Diseases, Kolkata** for extending all the facilities, valuable suggestions and help provided to carry out in-vitro *Helicobacter pylori* growth inhibition study.

I also express my sincere thanks to **Martina Bio Genics Private Limited,** Chowhati, Rajpur, Kolkata 700 151, for their kind support by giving the drug as gift sample.

I am extremely grateful to the **Head of the Department, Metallurgical Department, Jadavpur University** for his extreme help during SEM Study.

I would like to convey my gratitude to **Mr. Arnab De & Mr. Souvik Ojha**, who helped me lot during my thesis work.

I would like to express my special thanks to **Mr. Bhaskar Das,** my lab mate, for his co-operation during FTIR study.

I place on record my thanks to the authors of the books and research papers which I consulted during my work, I have acknowledged them in reference section of this thesis.

I am indeed glad to convey cordial thanks to all of my friends, relatives and labmates especially Anurup Mandal, Aditya Kumar Jena, Mousumi Das, Sayantani Das, Debmalya Mitra, Samit Bera and all others who have extended their co-operation to carry-out this work successfully.

Finally, I acknowledge with gratitude the help and support I received from my wife, **Sarmila** who suffered a lot to keep me free from social responsibilty enambling me to reach this stage today. I can never forget to appreciate little but loving help of my daughter, **Samadrita**.

Last but not the least; I dedicate the pleasure of presenting this thesis at the lotus feet of the almighty.

....

(Sanjoy Kumar Dey)

CONTENTS

Chapter I

INTRODUCTION

1.1. Introduction

The high level of patient compliance in taking oral dosage forms is due to the ease of administration and handling of these forms [1]. Development of a successful oral controlled release formulation requires an understanding of three aspects: (a) gastrointestinal physiology (b) physiochemical properties of the drug and (c) dosage form characteristics [2]. In the development of oral controlled drug delivery system, one of the main challenges is to modify the GI transit time [1]. Using controlled release technology, oral delivery for 24 h(hours) is possible for many drugs; however, the substance must be well absorbed throughout the whole gastrointestinal tract. A significant obstacle may arise if there is a narrow window for drug absorption in the gastro intestinal tract (GIT), if a stability problem exists in gastrointestinal fluids, or the drug is poorly soluble in the intestine or acts locally in the stomach. Thus, the real issue in the development of oral controlled release dosage forms is not just to prolong the delivery of the drugs for more than 12 h, but to prolong the presence of the dosage forms in the stomach or somewhere in the upper intestine until the entire drug is released over the desired period of time [3]. These considerations have led to the development of a unique oral controlled release dosage form with gastroretentive properties. Floating Drug Delivery System(FDDS) have a bulk density less than gastric fluids and so remain buoyant in the stomach without affecting gastric emptying rate for a prolonged period of time. After oral administration, such a dosage form would be retained in the stomach and release the drug there in a controlled and prolonged manner, so that the drug could be supplied continuously to its absorption sites in the upper gastrointestinal tract. This result in a better control of the fluctuations in plasma drug concentration and improves bioavailability, therapeutic efficacy and may even also allow a possible reduction in the dose because of steady therapeutic levels of different antimicrobials.

The reduction in fluctuations in therapeutic levels minimizes the risk of resistance especially in case of β-lactam antibiotics (penicillin's and cephalosporins) [4]. Gastroretentive floating dosage forms are also useful for local as well as sustained delivery of antimicrobials to treat *Helicobacter pylori (H. pylori)* infection which is the cause of peptic ulcers. In this project oil entrapped chitosan coated amoxicillin trihydrate floating beads were prepared by the emulsion gelation method and were evaluated for various parameters like size, weight variation, drug entrapment efficiency, in-vitro floating, in-vitro drug release, in-vitro *H. pylori* growth inhibition and in-vivo floating with the aim to localize the antibiotic at the site of *H. pylori* infection to achieve higher bactericidal concentration and thereby to improve the therapeutic efficacy of the drug.

1.2. Floating Drug Delivery System

Floating systems or dynamically controlled systems are low-density systems that have sufficiently buoyancy to float over the gastric contents and remain buoyant in the stomach without affecting the gastric emptying rate for a prolonged period of time (Fig:1.1).

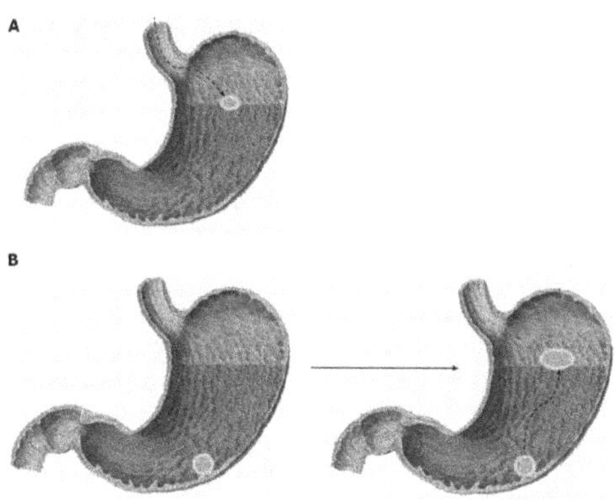

Fig. 1.1. Floating systems: Low-density floating dosage (A) and the density of dosage can be lowered after administration (B).

1.3. Advantages of Floating Drug Delivery System

- **Predictable drug release from dosage forms:** Majority of drugs are preferentially absorbed from the upper part of the small intestine. Floating drug delivery system has the advantage that after oral administration; dosage form would be retained in the stomach and releases the drug there in a controlled and prolonged manner, so that the drug could be supplied continuously to its absorption sites in the upper GIT.
- **Pharmacokinetic advantages:** As sustained release systems, floating dosage forms offer various potential advantages evident from several recent publications. Drugs that have poor bioavailability because their absorption is restricted to the upper GIT can be delivered efficiently thereby maximizing their absorption and improving their absolute bioavailability. e.g. Furosemide [5].
- **Reduces the gastric irritation:** Floating drug delivery is useful to reduce the gastric irritation caused by various non steroidal anti-inflammatory drugs.
- **Pharmacotherapy of the stomach:** Gastroretentive floating drug delivery greatly improves the pharmacotherapy of the stomach through local drug release resulting in high drug concentrations at the gastric mucosa [6]. e.g. Eradication of *H. pylori,* the causative agent of chronic dyspepsia, gastric and duodenal ulcer by Clarithromycin [7], Amoxicillin [8] etc.
- **Minimized adverse activity at the colon:** Retention of the drug in the stomach minimizes the amount of drug that reaches the colon. This pharmacodynamic aspect provides the rationale for gastroretentive formulations of beta-lactam antibiotics (penicillins and cephalosporins) [4] that are absorbed only from the small intestine and whose presence in the colon leads to the development of microorganism's resistance.

- **Absorption Enhancement:** A floating dosage form is feasible approach especially for drugs which have limited absorption site in stomach and upper small intestine. e.g. Frusemide [9], P-amino benzoic acid [10] etc.
- **Enhanced bioavailability:** There are some drugs such as Ofloxacin [11], Chlordiazepoxide, Diazepam, and Cinnarizine [12] etc which are poorly soluble at intestinal pH and dissolution is the rate limiting step in the absorption and bioavailability. Floating drug delivery of these drugs increases their bioavailability by reducing their wastage.
- **Enhanced first pass biotransformation:** In similar fashion to the increased efficacy of active transporters exhibiting capacity limited activity, the pre-systemic metabolism of the tested compound may be considerably increased when the drug is presented to the metabolic enzymes (cytochrome P450, in particular CYP3A4) in a sustained manner by FDDS, rather than by a bolus input.
- **Reduce fluctuation of drug concentration:** Continuous input of the drug following control release gastro retentive dosage form (GRDF) administration produces blood drug concentration within a narrower range compared to the immediate release dosage forms. Thus, fluctuation in drug effects is minimized and concentration dependent adverse effects that are associated with peak concentration can be prevented. This feature is of special importance for drugs with a narrow therapeutic index. [13]
- **Improved selectivity in receptor activation:** Minimization of fluctuation in drug concentration also makes it possible to obtain certain selectivity in the elicited pharmacological effect of drug that activates different type of receptors at different concentration.

1.4. Disadvantages of Floating Drug Delivery System

- There are certain situations where gastric retention is not desirable. Aspirin and non-steroidal anti-inflammatory drugs are known to cause gastric lesions, and slow release of such drugs in the stomach is unwanted.
- Drugs that may irritate the stomach lining or are unstable in its acidic environment should not be formulated in gastroretentive systems.
- Furthermore, some drugs, such as Isosorbide dinitrate, that are absorbed equally well throughout the GIT will not benefit from incorporation into a gastric retention system.

1.5. Mechanism of Floating Systems

Various attempts have been made to retain the dosage form in the stomach as a way of increasing the retention time. Floating drug delivery systems (FDDS) have a bulk density less than gastric fluids and so remain buoyant in the stomach without affecting the gastric emptying rate for a prolonged period of time. While the system is floating on the gastric contents (Fig.1.2.), the drug is released slowly at the desired rate from the system. After release of drug, the residual system is emptied from the stomach. This resulted in an increased gastric retention time (GRT) and a better control of the fluctuations of plasma drug concentration.

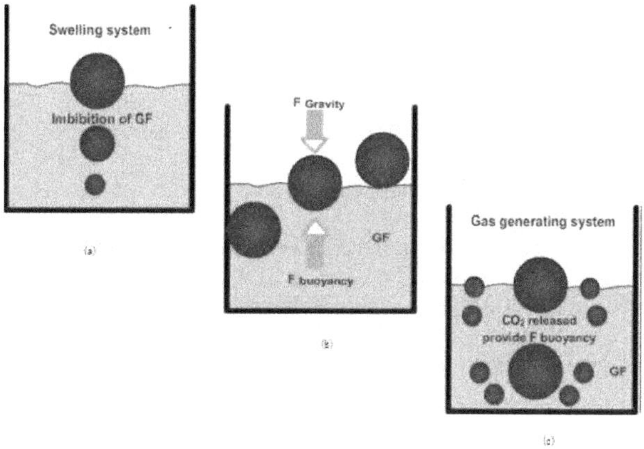

Fig. 1.2. Mechanism of floating system, GF= Gastric fluid.

However, besides a minimal gastric content needed to allow the proper achievement of the buoyancy retention principle, a minimal level of floating force (F) is also required to keep the dosage form reliably buoyant on the surface of the meal. To measure the floating force kinetics, a novel apparatus for determination of resultant weight has been reported in the literature. The apparatus operates by measuring continuously the force equivalent to F (as a function of time) that is required to maintain the submerged object. The object floats better if F is on the higher positive side (Fig. 1.2.). This apparatus helps in optimizing FDDS with respect to stability and durability of floating forces produced in order to prevent the drawbacks of unforeseeable intragastric buoyancy capability variations [14].

$F = F\ buoyancy - F\ gravity = (D_f - D_s)\ gv$

Where, F= total vertical force, D_f = fluid density, D_s = object density, v = volume and g = acceleration due to gravity.

1.6. Basic Gastrointestinal Tract Physiology

The GIT is essentially a tube about nine metres long that runs through the middle of the body from the mouth to the anus and includes the throat (pharynx), oesophagus, stomach, small intestine (consisting of the duodenum, jejunum and ileum) and large intestine (consisting of the cecum, appendix, colon and rectum). The stomach is an organ with a capacity for storage and mixing [15]. Anatomically (Fig.1.3.) the stomach is divided into 3 regions: fundus, body, and antrum (pylorus). The proximal part made of fundus and body acts as reservoir for undigested material, whereas the antrum is the main site for mixing motions and acts as a pump for gastric emptying by propelling action.

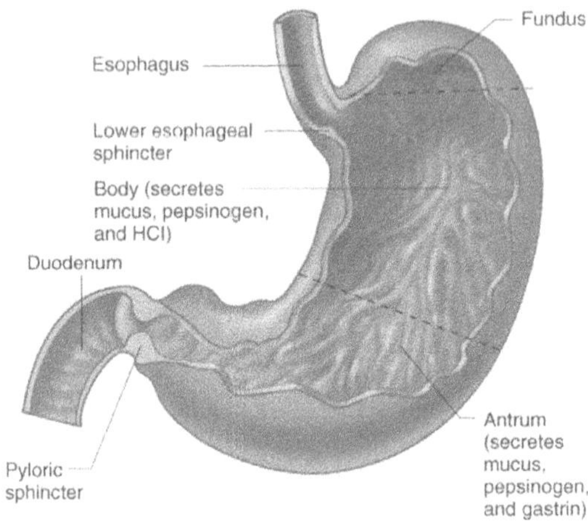

Fig. 1.3. Anatomy of human stomach.

Gastric emptying occurs during fasting as well as in fed states (Fig. 1.4). The pattern of motility is however distinct in the 2 states. During the fasting state an interdigestive series of electrical events take place, which cycle both through stomach and intestine every 2 to 3 h [16]. This is called the interdigestive myloelectric cycle or migrating myloelectric cycle (MMC), which is further divided into following 4 phases (Fig. 1.5) as described by Wilson and Washington [17].

1. Phase I (basal phase) lasts from 40 to 60 minutes with rare contractions.

2. Phase II (preburst phase) lasts for 40 to 60 minutes with intermittent action potential and contractions. As the phase progresses the intensity and frequency also increases gradually.

3. Phase III (burst phase) lasts for 4 to 6 minutes. It includes intense and regular contractions for short period. It is due to this wave that all the undigested material is swept out of the stomach down to the small intestine. It is also known as the housekeeper wave.

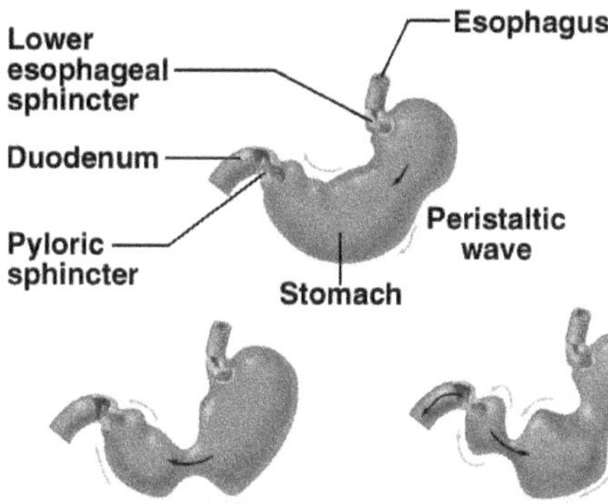

Fig 1.4. Waves of smooth muscle contraction mix and propel the ingested contents of the gastric lumen, but only a small amount of the material enters the small intestine (duodenum) as a result of each wave cycle.

4. Phase IV lasts for 0 to 5 minutes and occurs between phases III and I of 2 consecutive cycles.

After the ingestion of a mixed meal, the pattern of contractions changes from fasted to that of fed state. This is also known as digestive motility pattern and comprises continuous contractions as in phase II of fasted state. These contractions result in reducing the size of food particles (to less than 1 mm), which are propelled toward the pylorus in a suspension form. During the fed state onset of MMC is delayed resulting in slowdown of gastric emptying rate [16].

Scintigraphic studies determining gastric emptying rates revealed that orally administered controlled release dosage forms are subjected to basically 2 complications, that of short gastric residence time and unpredictable gastric emptying rate. The concentration of the hormone motilin in the blood controls the duration of the phases [18].

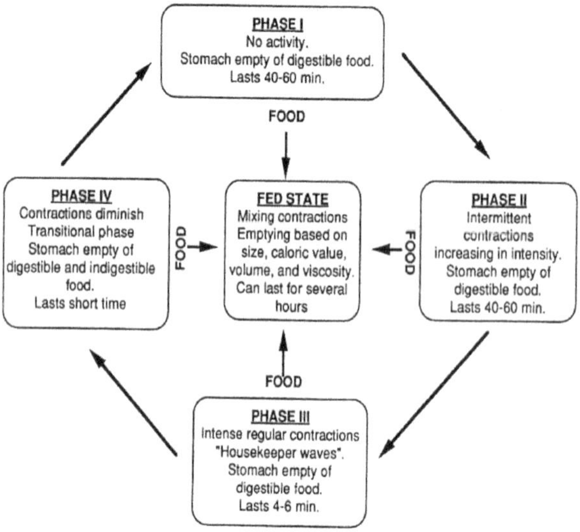

Fig. 1.5. Diagram showing the four phases of migrating myoelectric cycle.

1.7. Factors Controlling Gastric Retention of Dosage Forms

The floating time of dosage forms is controlled by several factors such as

- **Density of dosage form:** Density of the dosage form must be lower than the gastric fluids for showing the floating behavior. Normally a density of <1.0 gm/cm^3 is required to exhibit floating property.
- **Size of dosage form:** Dosage form units with a diameter of more than 9.5mm are reported to have an increased GRT.

- **Shape of dosage form:** It was reported that tetrahedron and ring shaped devices have a better gastric residence time as compared with other shapes.
- **Fed or unfed state:** Under fasting conditions, the gastro intestinal motility is characterized by periods of strong motor activity or the migrating myoelectric complex (MMC) that occurs every 2 to 3 h [19]. The MMC sweeps undigested materials from the stomach and if the timing of the formulation coincides with that of the MMC, the gastroretentive time of the dosage form can be expected to be very short. However, in the fed state, MMC is delayed resulting in slowdown of gastric empting rate [16].
- **Nature of meal:** Feeding of indigestible polymers or fatty acid salts can change the motility pattern of the stomach to a fed state, thus decreasing the gastric emptying rate and prolonging drug release.[20]
- **Caloric content and frequency of feed:** GRT can be increased with a meal that is high in proteins and fats and when successive meals are given compared with a single meal due to the low frequency of MMC.
- **Biological factors:** Biological factors such as age, body mass index, gender, posture, and diseased states (diabetes, Chron's disease) influence gastric emptying. In the case of elderly persons, especially those over 70, have a significantly longer GRT. Mean ambulatory GRT in males is less compared with their age and race-matched female counterparts, regardless of the weight, height and body surface. Generally females have slower gastric emptying rates than males. GRT also can vary between supine and upright ambulatory states of the patient [21]. Stress increases gastric emptying rates while depression slows it down [22].
- **Intake of drugs:** Anti-cholinergic and opiates increase the GRT [23] by decreasing the peristalsis where as prokinetics like Metoclopramide decrease the GRT by increasing peristalsis.

1.8. Suitable Drug Candidates for Floating Dosage Forms

Various drugs have their greatest therapeutic effect when released in the stomach, particularly when the release is prolonged in a continuous, controlled manner. Drugs delivered in this manner have a lower level of side effects and provide their therapeutic effects without the need for repeated dosages or with a low dosage frequency. Sustained release in the stomach is also useful for therapeutic agents that the stomach does not readily absorb, since sustained release prolongs the contact time of the agent in the stomach or in the upper part of the small intestine, which is where absorption occurs and contact time is limited. Under normal or average conditions, for example, material passes through the small intestine in as little as 1-3 h [24].

In general, appropriate candidates for floating drug delivery are molecules that have poor colonic absorption but are characterized by better absorption properties at the upper parts of the GIT:

- Narrow absorption window in GIT, e.g., Riboflavin and Levodopa.
- Primarily absorbed from stomach and upper part of GIT, e.g., Calcium supplements, Chlordiazepoxide and Cinnarazine.
- Drugs that act locally in the stomach, e.g., Antacids and Misoprostol.
- Drugs that degrade in the colon, e.g., Ranitidine HCl and Metronidazole.
- Low density form of the dosage forms that causes buoyancy in gastric fluid [25]
- High density dosage forms which are retained in the bottom of the stomach [26]
- Bioadhesion to stomach mucosa [27].
- Slowed motility of the gastrointestinal tract by concomitant administration of drugs or pharmaceutical excipients [28].

- Expansion by swelling or unfolding to a large size which limits emptying of the dosage form through the pyloric sphincter [29].

Table 1.1. Commonly used drugs in different type of floating dosage forms:

Dosage forms	Drugs
Tablets	Acetaminophen, Ampicillin, Amoxicillin trihydrate, Ciprofloxacin, Levofloxacin, Atenolol, Diltiazem.
Capsules	Clarithromycin, Celecoxib, Diazepam, Furosemide,
Beads	Amoxicillin, Clarithromycin, Ciprofloxacin, Levofloxacin hemihydrate.
Granules	Diclofenac sodium, Indomethacin, Gatifloxacin.
Microspheres	Amoxicillin, Cefopodoxim proxetil, Ciprofloxacin, Clarithromycin, Ofloxacin, Aspirin, Griseofulvin.
Nanoparticles	Amoxicillin
In Situ Gel	Levofloxacin hemihydrate.

Table 1.2. Available marketed gastroretentive formulations:

Brand name	Drug (dose)	Company, country	Type of formulation
Madopar	Levodopa(100 mg) Benserazide(25mg)	Roche product,USA	Floating CR capsule
Valrelease	Diazepam(15mg)	Hoffmann- LaRoche,USA	Floating capsule
Liquid gaviscon	$Al(OH)_2$ (95mg) MgCarbonate(385mg)	GSK, India	Effervescent floating liquid alginate preparation
cytotec	Misoprostal (100µgm/200 µgm)	Pharmaacia,USA	Bilayer floating capsule
Topalkan	Aluminum magnesium antacid	Pierre Fabre drug, France	Floating liquid alginate
Conviron	Ferrous sulfate	Ranbaxy, India	Gas generating floating form
Cifran OD	Ciprofloxacin(1gm)	Ranbaxy, India	Gas generating floating form

1.9. Polymers Used in Floating Drug Delivery Systems

Following types of ingredients can be used to prepare FDDS in addition to the drugs:

- Hydrocolloids (20%-75%): They can be synthetics, anionic or non-ionic like hydrophilic gums, modified cellulose derivatives. Eg. Acacia, Pectin, Chitosan, Agar, Casein, Bentonite, Veegum, HPMC (K4M, K100M and K15M), Gellan gum (Gelrite®), Sodium CMC, MC, HPC etc.
- Inert fatty materials(5%-75%): Edible, inert fatty materials having a specific gravity of less than one can be used to decrease the hydrophilic property of formulation and hence increase buoyancy. Eg. Beeswax, Sunflower oil, Soybean oil, Fatty acids, Long chain fatty alcohols, Gelucires® 39/01 and 43/01.
- Effervescent agents: Sodium bicarbonate, Citric acid, Tartaric acid, Di-Sodium Glycine Carbonate, Citroglycine etc.
- Release rate accelerants(5%-60%): eg Lactose, Mannitol
- Release rate retardants (5%-60%): eg Dicalcium phosphate, Talc, Magnesium stearate
- Buoyancy increasing agents (upto80%): eg. Ethyl cellulose
- Low density material: Polypropylene foam powder (Accurel MP 1000®).

1.10. Classification of Floating Drug Delivery Systems

Based on the formulation variables FDDS are classified into effervescent and non-effervescent systems.

A. Effervescent Floating Drug Delivery Systems:

These buoyant systems utilize matrices prepared with swellable polymers like Methocel®, Chitosan and various effervescent compounds like sodium bicarbonate, tartaric acid and citric acid. They are formulated in such-a-way that when in contact with the acidic gastric contents, carbondioxide is liberated and gets entrapped in swollen hydrocolloids, which provides buoyancy to the dosage forms (Fig. 1.6).

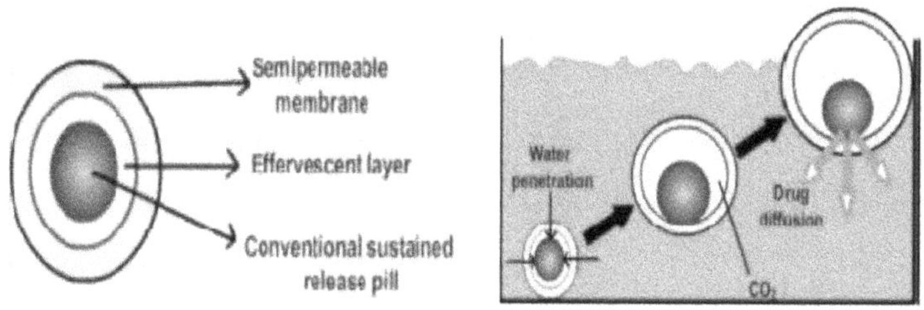

A B

Fig. 1.6. (A) Multiple unit oral FDDS, (B) Working principle of effervescent FDDS.

B. Non-effervescent Floating Drug Delivery System:

Non-effervescent floating drug delivery system use a gel forms or swellable cellulose type of hydrocolloids, polysaccharides and matrix forming polymers like polycarbonate, polyacrylate, polymethacrylate and polystyrene. Here floating property is achieved by following two mechanisms:

- The dosage form swells when it comes in contact with gastric fluids and attains a bulk density less than 1, the air entrapped within the swollen matrix imparts buoyancy to the dosage form. The soformed swollen gel-like structure acts as a reservoir and allows sustained release of drug through the gelatinous mass. Ex: Floating tablet.
- The inherent low density of dosage form helps in the buoyancy of the dosage form. Ex: Microporous compartment system.

This system can be further divided into four sub types:

I. Microporous Compartment System:

This technology is based on the encapsulation of a drug reservoir inside a microporous compartment with pores along its top and bottom walls. The peripheral walls of the drug reservoir compartment are completely sealed to prevent any direct contact of gastric surface with the undissolved drug. In the stomach, the floatation chamber containing entrapped air causes the delivery system to float over the gastric content. Gastric fluid enters through the aperture, dissolves the drug and carries the dissolved drug for continuous transport across the intestine for absorption.

II. Colloidal Gel Barrier System:

This system incorporates a high level of one or more gel forming cellulose type hydrocolloid e.g. hydroxypropyl cellulose, hydroxyethyl cellulose, hydroxypropyl methyl cellulose (HPMC), polysaccharides and matrix-forming polymer such as polycarbophil, polyacrylate and polystyrene. On coming in contact with gastric fluid, the hydrocolloid in the system swells and forms a colloid gel barrier around its surface maintaining its shape (Fig. 1.7). The air trapped by the swollen polymer confers the buoyancy of the dosage form and a bulk density less than unity. The gel barrier controls the rate of diffusion of solvent - in and drug out of the dosage form. They are formulated as tablet or capsule.

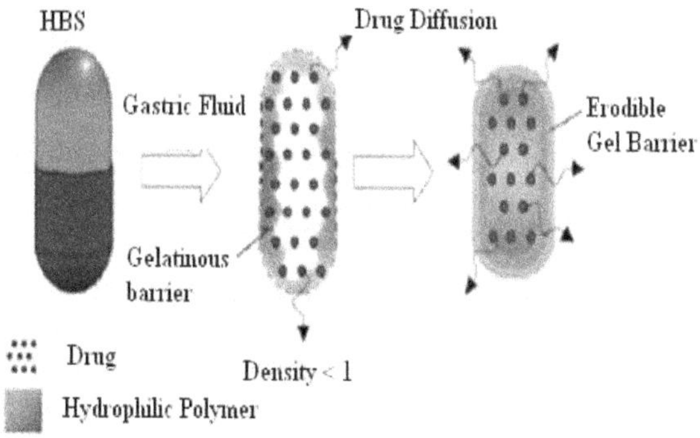

Fig. 1.7. Working principle of hydro dynamically balanced system.

III. Alginate Beads:

Multi-unit floating spherical floating beads of approximately 1.5 mm to 2.5 mm diameter can be prepared by dropping sodium alginate solution into aqueous solution of calcium chloride. Spherical gel beads formed instantaneously due to intermolecular cross linking between the divalent calcium ions and the negatively charged carboxyl group of alginic acid provided a gel barrier at the surface of the formulation. The beads are then separated, dried at 40°C. These beads when administered absorb gastro intestinal fluid and swell decreasing it's density and hence get floated (Fig. 1.8).

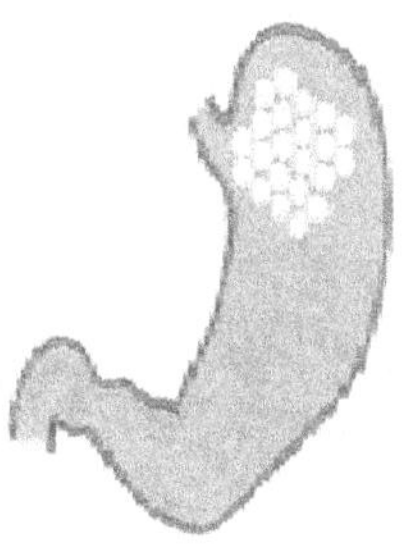

Fig. 1.8. Figure showing floating of alginate beads.

IV. Hollow Microspheres/ Microballons:

Hollow microspheres loaded with drug in their outer polymer shelf were prepared by a novel emulsion solvent diffusion method [30]. The ethanol/dichloromethane solution of the drug and an enteric acrylic polymer was poured into an agitated solution of Poly Vinyl Alcohol (PVA) that was thermally controlled at 40°C The gas phase is generated in the dispersed polymer droplet by the evaporation of dichloromethane forming an internal cavity in the microsphere of the polymer with drug (Fig. 1.9). The microballoon floated continuously over the surface of an acidic dissolution media containing surfactant for more than 12 h.

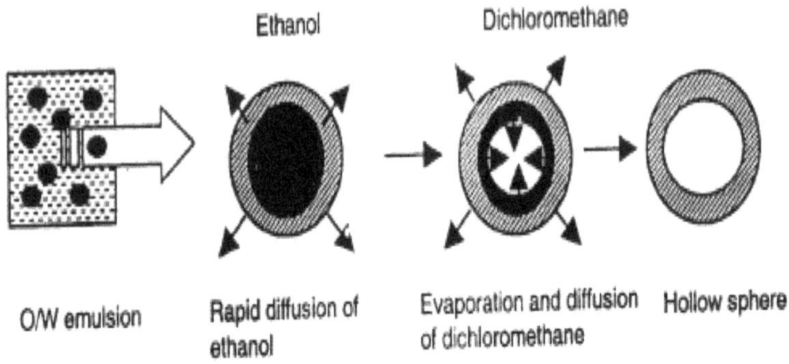

Fig1.9. Figure showing mechanism of formation of microballon.

1.11. Mechanism of Drug Release from Beads

The mechanism of drug release from beads can be occurring in the following ways:

a) **Diffusion:** On contact with aqueous fluids in the GIT, water diffuses into the interior of the bead. Drug dissolution occurs and the drug solutions diffuse across the gel barrier to the exterior.

b) Erosion: Some coating can be designed to erode gradually with time, thereby releasing the drug contained within the bead.

c) Osmosis: In allowing water to enter under the right circumstances, an osmotic pressure can be built up within the interior of the bead. The drug is forced out of the bead into the exterior through the coating.

1.12. Literature Review

Floating Tablets:

Pandit et al [31] prepared gastro retentive floating tablets of amoxicillin trihydrate using various grades of HPMC with the objective to obtain site-specific drug delivery and to extend its duration of action. Optimized formulation of amoxicillin was found to have increased gastric residence prolonging the release of drug with 85% of drug release in 6 h by diffusion. The mechanism of drug release was found to be diffusion and followed combination of zero order and first order kinetics.

Yin et al [32] developed gastrofloating tablets of cephalexin to prolong the residence time in major absorption sites. Gastro-floating tablets were prepared and optimized using hydroxypropyl methylcellulose (HPMC K100M) as matrix and sodium bicarbonate as a gas-forming agent. The properties of the tablets in terms of floating lag time, floating time and in-vitro release were evaluated. Furthermore, in-vivo pharmacokinetic study in fed and fasted beagle dogs was performed. The gastro-floating tablets had short floating lag time and exhibited a satisfactory sustained-release profile in-vitro. Compared with conventional capsules, the gastro-floating tablets presented a sustained-release behavior with a relative bioavailability of 99.4%, while the reference sustained-release tablets gave a relative bioavailability of only 39.3%. Meanwhile, the food had significant effect on the pharmacokinetics of sustained-release tablets. It was concluded that the gastro-floating tablets had a sustained-release effect in-vitro and in-vivo, as well as desired pharmacokinetic properties in both fed and fasted conditions.

Arza et al [33] developed swellable, floating, and sustained release tablets of ciprofloxacin by using a combination of hydrophilic polymer (hydroxypropyl methylcellulose), swelling agents (crospovidone, sodium starch glycolate, and croscarmelose sodium) and effervescent substance (sodium bicarbonate). Formulations are evaluated for percentage swelling, in-vitro drug release, floating lag time, total duration of floating, and mean residence time (MRT) in the stomach. In-vivo nature of thc tablet at different time intervals is observed in the radiographic pictures of the healthy volunteers and MRT in the stomach is found to be 320±48.99 min (n=6). A combination of HPMC K100M, crospovidone, and sodium carbonate shows the good swelling, drug release, and floating characters than the marketed CIFRAN OD®.

Patel et al [34] designed floating matrix tablets of clarithromycin to prolong the gastric residence time after oral administration, at a particular site and controlling the release of drug especially useful for achieving controlled plasma level as well as improving bioavailability. Floating tablets of clarithromycin containing HPMC and different additives were compressed using wet granulation and D-optimal design technique. The study shows that tablet composition and mechanical strength have great influence on the floating properties and drug release. Incorporation of gas-generating agent together with polymer improved drug release, besides optimal floating (floating lag time <30 s; total floating time >10 h). The drug release was sufficiently sustained (more than 8 h) and anomalous diffusion as well as zero-order was confirmed. The optimized formulation was obtained using 62.5% clarithromycin, 4.95% HPMC

K15M, 18.09% HPMC K4M, 12.96% sodium bicarbonate which gave floating lag time < 30 s with a total floating time > 10 h.

Bomma et al [35] developed floating matrix tablets of norfloxacin to prolong gastric residence time, leading to an increase in drug bioavailability. Tablets were prepared by the wet granulation technique, using polymers such as HPMC (HPMC K4M, HPMC K100M) and xanthan gum. The tablets exhibited controlled and prolonged drug release profiles while floating over the dissolution medium. In-vivo radiographic studies revealed that the tablets remained in the stomach for 180 ± 30 min in fasting human volunteers and indicated that gastric retention time was increased by the floating principle, which was considered desirable for the absorption window drugs.

Chavanpatil et al [36] Developed a new gastroretentive sustained release delivery system with floating, swellable and bioadhesive properties for ofloxacin using various release retarding polymers like psyllium husk, HPMC K100M and a swelling agent, crosspovidone. Formulations were evaluated for in-vitro drug release profile, swelling characteristics and in-vitro bioadhesion property. The in-vitro drug release followed Higuchi kinetics and the drug release mechanism was found to be of anomalous or non-Fickian type. The similarity factor $f2$ was found to be 91.12 for the developed formulation indicating the release was similar to that of the marketed formulation (Zanocin OD). The swelling properties were increased with increasing crosspovidone concentration and contributed significantly in drug release from the tablet matrix. The bioadhesive property of the developed formulation was found to be significant ($P < 0.005$) in combination as compared to HPMC K100M and psyllium husk alone.

Yang et al [37] proposed a new strategy for the triple drug treatment (tetracycline, metronidazole and bismuth salt) of *H. pylori* associated peptic ulcers. The design of the delivery system was based on the swellable asymmetric triple layer tablet approach, with floating feature in order to prolong the gastric retention time of the delivery system. Hydroxypropyl methylcellulose and poly (ethylene oxide) were the major rate-controlling polymeric excipients. Tetracycline and metronidazole were incorporated into the core layer of the triple-layer matrix for controlled delivery, while bismuth salt could be included in one of the outer layers for instant release. Results demonstrated that sustained delivery of tetracycline and metronidazole over 6–8 h can be easily achieved while the tablet remained afloat. The floating aspect was envisaged to extend the gastric retention time of the designed system to maintain effective localized concentration of tetracycline and metronidazole. Authors concluded that the developed delivery system has potential to increase the efficacy of the therapy and improve patient compliance.

Floating Capsules:

A new peroral amoxicillin/clavulanate therapeutic system composed of immediate release tablet and controlled release floating capsule was developed and evaluated by in-vivo bioavailability study by Kerč and Opara [38]. Pharmacokinetic (PK) parameters for amoxicillin and clavulanic acid of the new therapeutic systems: AUCt, AUCi, (AUCt/AUCi), Cmax, Tmax, kel, T1/2 and additionally for amoxicillin T_4 and T_2 were calculated from the plasma levels. The study confirmed enhanced pharmacokinetic parameters of a newly developed therapeutic system containing 1500 mg of amoxicillin and 125 mg of clavulanic acid. Prolonged time over MIC(minimum inhibitory concentration) of amoxicillin in relation to a regular immediate release amoxicillin/clavulanate formulation was also confirmed.

Neb et al [39] developed hydrodynamically balanced capsules of clarithromycin to prolong gastric residence time with the desired in-vitro release profile for the localized action in the stomach, in the treatment of *H. pylori* mediated peptic ulcer. HPMC K4M and Carbopol 934 were selected as release modifier polymeric fillers and sodium bicarbonate as the float accelerator. The capsules were prepared by physical blending of clarithromycin and the polymer in varying ratios. Incorporation of gasgenerating agent together with polymer improved drug release, besides optimal floating. A 3^2 factorial design was applied to study the effect of individual formulation variables on the final formulation and their interaction with each other. The formulation developed using 30% HPMC K4M polymer and 10% sodium bicarbonate showed promising responses with respect to n, t50, t85 and Q12.

Floating Beads:

Sahasathian et al [40] formulated chitosan-coated mucoadhesive floating alginate beads as a gastroretensive delivery vehicle for amoxicillin, towards the effective eradication of *H. pylori*, a major causative agent of peptic ulcers. Amoxicillin loaded alginate beads coated with 0.5% (w/v) chitosan exhibited excellent floating ability, high encapsulation efficiency, high drug loading capacity, sustained release of amoxicillin for over six hours in simulated gastric fluid and a strong in-vitro mucoadhesion to the gastric mucosal layer.

Fursule et al [41] described the formulation and evaluation of gastroretentive system of an antibacterial agent, amoxicillin trihydrate, based on the concept of altered density. Different formulations of oil entrapped floating gel beads were prepared by using sodium alginate as gelling agent. The prepared beads were evaluated for diameter, surface morphology and encapsulation efficiency. Authors concluded that the oil entrapped gel beads can be used as FDDS for local as well as systemic drug delivery.

Nimase et al [42] prepared multiple-unit floating beads of clarithromycin containing sodium alginate hydroxypropyl methylcellulose (K100M) and sunflower oil using the technique of three variables at three levels (3^3) factorial design. Total twenty-seven possible batches were prepared and were evaluated for entrapment efficiency, drug loading, buoyancy and in-vitro drug release. All formulations showed floating lag time below 2 minutes and showed total floating duration more than 10 h. The release rate, entrapment efficiency, drug loading and buoyancy was greater with formulation containing 2 percent sodium alginate solution and 5 percent calcium chloride solution along with 5 ml sunflower oil.

Gattani et al [43] developed alginate/HPMC based floating-mucoadhesive beads of clarithromycin to provide prolonged contact time of antibiotic to treat stomach ulcer. Beads were prepared by ionic gelation technique where calcium chloride used as gelating agent and incorporated liquid paraffin for floating of the beads. Prepared beads were evaluated extensively for particle size, drug entrapment; swelling and surface morphology by using scanning electron microscopy. X-ray radioimaging study in rabbits, in-vitro mucoadhesion using rat stomach mucosal membrane and in-vitro drug release studies were carried out. Ex-vivo performance of alginate-HPMC beads were studied using albino rats in comparison to simple alginate-calcium beads. Authors concluded that alginate-HPMC beads may be suitable floating-muco-adhesive drug delivery system for delivering clarithromycin to treat stomach ulcers.

Srinatha et al [44] prepared chitosan beads loaded with ciprofloxacin hydrochloride and fabricated by ionic cross-linking with sodium tripolyphosphate. Authors found that minimum curing time is important for high drug loading. Authors also found that drug release increased with higher concentration of drug in decreasing proportion of chitosan.

Floating Granules:

Shah et al [45] prepared controlled-release multiunit floating lipid granules of gatifloxacin using Gelucire 39/01, and Gelucire 43/01 by the melt granulation technique and evaluated for in-vitro floating and drug release. Ethyl cellulose was taken as release rate modifier. Authors found that moderate amount of Gelucire 39/01 and ethyl cellulose provides desired release of gatifloxacin from a floating system. The temperature sensitivity studies for the prepared formulations at 40°C/75% relative humidity for 3 months showed no significant change in in-vitro drug release pattern.

Floating Micro Particles:

Patel et al [46] prepared mucoadhesive amoxicillin microspheres by simple emulsification phase separation technique using glutaraldehyde as a cross-linking agent and chitosan as mucoadhesive polymer. In-vitro mucoadhesive test showed that amoxicillin mucoadhesive microspheres adhered more strongly to gastric mucous layer and could retain in gastrointestinal tract for an extended period of time. The best batch exhibited a high drug entrapment efficiency of 70% and a swelling index of 1.39; percentage mucoadhesion after 1 h was 79 %. The drug release was also sustained for more than 12 h. Results of in-vivo *H. pylori* clearance tests on Wistar rats showed that amoxicillin mucoadhesive microspheres had a better clearance effect than amoxicillin powder. Authors concluded that the prolonged gastrointestinal residence time and enhanced amoxicillin stability resulting from the mucoadhesive microspheres of amoxicillin might make contribution complete eradication of *H. pylori*.

Cuna et al [47] prepared microparticles of amoxicillin-loaded ion-exchange resin encapsulated in polycarbophil and Carbopol 934 mucoadhesive polymers by modified oil-in-oil solvent evaporation technique. The prepared microspheres were evaluated for morphology and size, drug release, drug content and gastric transit time in rats. Polycarbophil microparticles were spherical, while carbopol 934 microparticles were irregular. In-vitro release of amoxicillin was rapid with or without a polymer coating. However, the gastrointestinal transit time was longer, and the distribution of the particles on the mucosa apparently better, without any polymer coating. Therefore, the authors concluded that microencapsulation of ion-exchange resin particles in the mucoadhesive polymers polycarbophil and Carbopol 934 failed to prolong their residence in the stomach of rats to a significant extent and appeared to favour the aggregation of the particles thereby making the distribution of particles in the stomach more difficult.

Nagahara et al [48] formulated amoxicillin in the form of mucoadhesive microspheres by spray chilling method, which have the ability to reside in the gastrointestinal tract for an extended period. The microspheres contained the amoxicillin and carboxyvinyl and curdlan as adhesive polymers dispersed in melted hydrogenated castor oil. The prepared microspheres were compared to 0.5% methylcellulose amoxicillin suspension in infected Mongolian gerbils under feeding conditions. The percentage of amoxicillin remaining in the stomach both 2 and 4 h after oral administration of the mucoadhesive microspheres was about three times higher than that after administration in the form of a 0.5% methylcellulose suspension. Both formulations showed anti *H. pylori* effects, with effective reduction of the required dose of amoxicillin by a factor of 10 when the mucoadhesive microspheres were used.

Karthikeyan et al [49] studied effect of different grades of HPMC on cefpodoxime proxetil release profile from floating microspheres. The cefpodoxime proxetil microspheres were prepared by non aqueous solvent evaporation method using HPMC K15M(15cps), HPMCK4M(4000cps), HPMC100LV(100cps) and ethyl cellulose. The prepared floating microspheres were found to produce the percentage yield of 50.5-72.21%, drug entrapment efficiency of 14.1-28.2%, buoyancy percentage of 70.1-88.25% and drug release of 65.09-101.88%. The better drug release profile was found to be formulation with drug : polymer ratio of 1:2 and HPMC 15cps showed much significant increase in the drug release while comparing with the other two grades of HPMC.

Deepa et al [50] prepared floating microspheres of cefpodoxime proxetil in order to achieve an extended retention in the upper GIT, which may result in enhanced absorption and thereby improved bioavailability. The microspheres were prepared by non-aqueous solvent evaporation method using polymers such as HPMC K15M, ethyl cellulose in different ratios and cefpodoxime proxetil in each formulation. The yield, particle size, buoyancy percentage, drug entrapment efficiency, and in-vitro drug release were studied. The result showed that microspheres yielded 50.5-72.2%, particle size was 75-600 μm, drug entrapment efficiency was 14.1-28.2%, and buoyancy percentage was 70.1-88.3%. The best drug release profiles were seen with formulation having the ratio of drug to polymer of 1:2.

Sarojini et al [51] developed albumin-chitosan based floating mucoadhesive microsphere of clarithromycin to provide prolonged contact time for drug delivery of antibiotics to treat stomach ulcers, increase the gastric residence time, decrease the diffusional distance, and also act locally at the infectious site. Microspheres prepared by heat stabilization method in the presence of span-80 were optimized by varying different formulation and processes parameters like drug to polymer ratio. It was subjected to evaluation for particle size, incorporation efficiency, in-vitro buoyancy and in-vitro drug release. Drug release from microsphere was found to be first order. It was concluded that drug-loaded microsphere appear to be a suitable delivery system for clarithromycin.

Venkateswaramurthy et al [52] developed controlled release mucoadhesive microspheres of amoxicillin trihydrate for the treatment of peptic ulcer disease caused by *H. pylori.* Microspheres were prepared by solvent evaporation technique using carbopol 974P, hydroxypropyl methyl cellulose K4M (HPMC K4M) and Eudragit RS 100 and were subjected to evaluation for particle size, incorporation efficiency, in-vitro mucoadhesion and in-vitro drug release characteristics. The prepared microspheres showed a strong mucoadhesive property. The polymer concentration influenced the in-vitro drug release significantly in 0.1N HCl. The particle sizes of systems ranged between 123±8.35 μm and 524±11.54 μm. The percentage drug entrapment and percentage yield of formulations were about 56.71±1.66% to 88.32±0.65% and 39.20±1.62% to 92.40±1.32%, respectively. The stability of the drugs was assessed in 0.1 N HCl. The results further substantiated that mucoadhesive microspheres improved the gastric stability of amoxicillin trihydrate (due to entrapment within the microsphere).

Sahoo et al [53] developed floating microspheres of ciprofloxacin hydrochloride by simple dripping method using a polymer mixture of sodium alginate and hydroxyl propyl methyl cellulose and sodium bicarbonate as gas forming agent. The prepared floating microspheres were evaluated for particle size distribution, floating behavior, drug content and in-vitro drug release. The prepared microspheres showed enhanced buoyancy and controlled release of the drug.

Floating Nanoparticles:

A novel hydrogel nanoparticles containing amoxicillin were synthesized by Moogooee et al [54]. The drug loaded hydrogel nanoparticles were prepared using the mucoadhesive polymer cross-linked N-isopropylacrylamide-acrylic acid-hydroxyethyl methacrylate. The prepared nanoparticles were characterized for their entrapment efficiency, mean diameter, morphology and in-vitro release in both pH 1.0 and 7.4 media. It was found that about 88.5% of amoxicillin entrapped in the nanoparticles was released in 4 h in the pH 1.0 medium, whereas in phosphate buffer at pH 7.4 not more than 45% was released after 4 h of dissolution study. In-vivo studies were performed to determine the drug concentration in rats' gastric tissues. The studies revealed that the hydrogel nanoparticles enhance drug concentration at gastric site than powder amoxicillin. Thus, the authors concluded that the developed hydrogel nanoparticle formulation may provide therapeutic concentration at a much lower dose that may reduce the adverse effects of amoxicillin in high doses.

In-Situ Floating Gels:

Mishra et al [55] prepared floating in situ gelling system of clarithromycin (FIGC) using gellan as gelling polymer and calcium carbonate as floating agent for potentially treating gastric ulcers, associated with *H. pylori*. Gellan based FIGC was prepared by dissolving varying concentrations of gellan in deionized water to which varying concentrations of drug and sucralfate were dispersed well. The formulation parameters like concentrations of gellan gum and sucralfate influenced the rate and extent of in-vitro drug release significantly from FIGC. The addition of sucralfate to the formulation significantly suppressed the degradation of clarithromycin at low pH. The in-vivo *H. pylori* clearance efficacy of prepared FIGC and clarithromycin suspension following oral administration, to *H. pylori* infected Mongolian gerbils was examined by polymerase chain reaction (PCR) technique and by a microbial culture method. FIGC showed a significant anti-*H. pylori* effect than that of clarithromycin suspension. The in situ gel formulation with sucralfate cleared *H. pylori* more effectively than that of formulation without sucralfate. In addition, the required amount of clarithromycin for eradication of *H. pylori* was found to be less from FIGC than from the corresponding clarithromycin suspension. It was concluded that prolonged gastrointestinal residence time and enhanced clarithromycin stability resulting from the floating in situ gel of clarithromycin might contribute better for complete clearance of *H. pylori*.

A gellan based floating in situ gelling system for controlled delivery of amoxicillin was developed by Rajinikanth et al [56]. The systems were prepared by dissolving varying concentrations of gellan gum in deionized water containing sodium citrate, to which varying concentrations of drug and calcium carbonate, as gas-forming agent, was added and dissolved by stirring. The in-vivo *H. pylori* clearance efficacy of prepared amoxicillin floating in situ gelling system (AFIG) was studied in *H. pylori* infected Mongolian gerbils following repeated oral administration by polymerase chain reaction technique and by a microbial culture method in comparison to amoxicillin suspension. The AFIG showed a significant anti- *H. pylori*, where the required amount of amoxicillin for eradication of *H. pylori* was 10 times less than that from the corresponding amoxicillin suspension.

1.13. Conclusion

FDDS is a novel drug delivery system which is so far limited to the experimental works, but system is having lot of prospective. In present era, therapeutic efficacy is a major issue in front of formulation and development pharmacists. In such situation FDDS will play an important role. FDDS reduces the fluctuations in the plasma level of antimicrobials delaying their gastric emptying. Antimicrobials that have poor bioavailability because of their limited absorption to the upper gastrointestinal tract or low bioavailability due to extensive first pass metabolism or have a local action in stomach can be delivered efficiently by FDDS thereby improving their therapeutic efficacy.

1.14. References

[1] Y.W Chien, Novel drug delivery systems, 2nd ed., Marcel Dekker, Inc., New York 1992.

[2] C.G. Wilson, N. Washington., Physiological Pharmaceutics: Biological Barriers to Drug Absorption, Horwood Ellis, Chichester, 1989, pp. 47-70.

[3] S. Baumgartner, J. Kristl, F. Vrecer, P. Vodopivec, B. Zorko, Optimization of floating matrix tablets and evaluation of their gastric residence time. Int. J. Pharm. 195 (2000) 125–135.

[4] B.M. Singh, K.H. Kim, Floating drug delivery systems: an approach to controlled drug delivery via gastric retention. J. Controlled Release. 63(3) (2000) 235–259.

[5] A. Menon, W.A. Ritschel, A. Sakr, Development and evaluation of a monolithic floating dosage form for furosemide. J. Pharm. Sci. 83(2) (1994) 239-245.

[6] A. Sayeed, M.B. Kinagi, M.H. Mohiuddin, S. Gada, S.M. Noorulla, Gastro retentive drug delivery systems: a review, Der Pharmacia Lettre. 3(1) (2011) 121-137.

[7] P.S. Rajinikanth, B. Mishra, Floating in situ gelling system for stomach site-specific delivery of clarithromycin to eradicate *H. pylori*, J. Controlled Release. 125(1) (2008) 33-41.

[8] L. Whitehead, J.H. Collett, J.T. Fell, Amoxicillin release from a floating dosage form based on Alginates. Int. J. Pharm. 210 (2000) 45–49.

[9] R. Bera, B. Mandal, M. Bhowmik, H. Bera, S.K. Dey, G. Nandi, L.K. Ghosh, Formulation and in-vitro evaluation of sunflower oil entrapped within buoyant beads of furosemide. Sci. Pharm. 77 (2009) 669–678.

[10] M. Ichikawa, T. Kato, M. Kawahara, S. Watanabe, M. Kayano, A New multiple-unit oral floating dosage system II: In-vivo evaluation of floating and sustained release characteristics with p-amino benzoic acid and Isosorbide di nitrate as model drugs. J. Pharm. Sci. 80(12) (1991) 1153-1156.

[11] D. Janardhan, J. Sreekanth, V. Bharat, P.R. Subramaniyan, Formulation and evaluation of gastro retentive drug delivery system for ofloxacin. Int. J. Pharm. Sci. Nanotechnol. 2(1) (2009) 428-434.

[12] H.N. Shivakumar, B.G. Desai, M. Patel, Optimization of gastroretentive system for oral controlled delivery of cinnarizine using response surface methodology. Ars Pharm. 48 (1) (2007) 55-81.

[13] A. Hoffman, Pharmacodynamic aspects of sustained release preparation. Adv. Drug Delivery Rev. 33(3) (1998) 185-199.

[14] S. Garg, S. Sharma, Gatroretentive drug delivery system in: Drug delivery oral, Business Briefing: Pharmatech, 2003, pp. 160-166.

[15] S. Desai, S. Bolton, A floating controlled released drug delivery system: In vitro-in vivo evaluation. Pharm. Res. 10(9) (1993) 1321-1325.

[16] G.R. Vantrappen, T.L. Peeters, J. Janssens, The secretory compartment of interdigestive migratory motor complex in man. Scand. J. Gastroenterol. 14(6) (1979) 663-667.

[17] C.G. Wilson, N. Washington., The stomach: its role in oral drug delivery, in: M.H. Rubinstein (eds.), Physiological Pharmaceutical: Biological Barriers to Drug Absorption, Chichester, UK: Ellis Horwood, 1989, pp. 47-70.

[18] J. Timmermans, A.J. Moes. How well do floating dosage forms float? Int. J. Pharm. 62 (1990) 207-216.

[19] G.R. Vantrappen, T.L. Peeters, J. Janssens, The secretory component of interdigestive migratory motor complex in man. Scand. J. Gastroenterol. 14(6) (1979) 663-667.

[20] A.J. Moes, Gastroretentive dosage forms, Crit. Rev. Ther. Drug Carrier Syst. 10(2) (1993) 193-195.

[21] L.J. Caldwell, R.C. Gardner, R.C. Cargill, Drug delivery device which can be retained in the stomach for a controlled period of time. US Patent 1998; 30th August: 4, 767, 627.

[22] B.N. Singh, K.H. Kim, Floating drug delivery systems: an approach to oral controlled drug delivery via gastric retention. J. Controlled Release. 63(3) (2000) 235-259.

[23] B.V. Gansbeke, J. Timmermans, A. Schoutens, A.J. Moes, Intragastric positioning of two concurrently ingested pharmaceutical matrix dosage forms. Nucl. Med. Biol. 18 (1991)711-718.

[24] F.N. Khan, M.G. Dehghan. Gastroretentive Drug Delivery Systems: A Patent Perspective, Int. J. Health. Res. 2009; 2(1): 23-44.

[25] A.A. Deshpande, N.H. Shah, C.T. Rhodes, W. Malick, Development of a novel controlled-release system for gastric retention. Pharm Res. 14(6) (1997) 815-819.

[26] S.S. Davis, A.F. Stockwell, M.J. Taylor, J.G. Hardy, D.R. Whalley, C.G. Wilson, H. Bechgaard, F.N. Christensen, The effect of density on the gastric emptying of single- and multiple-unit dosage forms. Pharm Res. 3(4) (1986) 208-213.

[27] C.M. Lehr, Bioadhesion technologies for the delivery of peptide and protein drugs to the gastrointestinal tract, Crit. Rev. Ther. Drug Carrier Syst. 11 (1994) 119-160.

[28] R. Groning, G. Heun, Oral dosage forms with controlled gastrointestinal transit, Drug Dev. Ind. Pharm. 10 (1984) 527-539.

[29] E.A. Klausner, E. Lavy, M. Friedman, A. Hoffman, Expandable gastroretentive dosage forms, J. Controlled Release. 90 (2003) 143-162.

[30] Y. Kawashinia, T. Niwa, H. Takcuchi, T. Hino, Y. Itoh, Hallow microspheres for use as a floating controlled drug delivery system in the stomach. J. Pharm. Sci. 81(2) (1992) 135-140.

[31] V. Pandit, S. Suresh, H. Joshi, Gastroretentive drug delivery system of amoxicillin: formulation and in-vitro evaluation, Int. J. Pharma Bio Sci. 1 (2010) 1-10.

[32] L. Yina, C. Qin, K. Chen, C. Zhu, H. Cao, J. Zhou, W. He, Q. Zhang, Gastro-floating tablets of cephalexin: Preparation and in-vitro/in-vivo evaluation, Int. J. Pharm. 452 (2013) 241–248.

[33] R.A.K. Arza, C.S.R. Gonugunta, P.R. Veerareddy, Formulation and evaluation of swellable and floating gastroretentive ciprofloxacin hydrochloride tablets, AAPS PharmSciTech. 10(1) (2009) 220-226.

[34] S.S. Patel, S. Ray, R.S. Thakur, Formualtion and evaluation of floating drug delivery system containing clarithromycin for *Helicobacter Pylori,* Acta Pol. Pharm. 63(1) (2006) 53-61.

[35] R. Bomma, R.A. Swamy Naidu, M.R. Yamsani, K. Veerabrahma, Development and evaluation of gastroretentive norfloxacin floating tablets, Acta Pharm. 59 (2009) 211–221.

[36] M.D. Chavanpatil, P. Jain, S. Chaudhari, R. Shear, P.R. Vavia, Novel sustained release, swellable and bioadhesive gastroretentivedrug delivery system for ofloxacin, Int. J. Pharm. 316 (2006) 86–92.

[37] L. Yang, J. Eshraghi, R. Fassihi, A new intragastric delivery system for the treatment of *Helicobacter pylori* associated gastric ulcer: in-vitro evaluation, J. Controlled Release. 57 (1999) 215-222.

[38] J. Kerč, J. Opara, A new Amoxicillin/clavulanate therapeutic system: preparation, in-vitro and pharmacokinetic evaluation, Int. J. Pharm. 335 (2007) 106-113.

[39] G.B. Neb, S.C. Atram, Y.K. Udavant, R.J. Salunke, S.R. Shahi, B.S. Gulecha, A.N. Padalkar, Formulation and evaluation of floating capsules of clarithromycin, J. Pharm. Res. 2(8) 2009 1348-1356.

[40] T. Sahasathian, N. Praphairaksit, N. Muangsin, Mucoadhesive and floating chitosan-coated alginate beads for the controlled gastric release of amoxicillin, Arch. Pharmacal Res. 33(6) (2010) 889-899.

[41] R.A. Fursule, CH.N. Patra, G.B.Patil, S.B. Kosalge, P.O. Patil, P.K. Deshmukh, Study of multiparticulate floating drug delivery system prepared by emulsion gelation technique, Int. J. ChemTech Res. 1 (2009) 162-167.

[42] P.K. Nimase, G. Vidyasagar, Preparation and evaluation of floating calcium alginate beads of Clarithromycin, Der Pharmacia Sinica. 1(1) (2010) 29-35.

[43] S.G. Gattani, P.J. Savaliya, V.S. Belgamwar, Floating-mucoadhesive beads of clarithromycin for the treatment of *Helicobacter pylori* infection, Chem. Pharm. Bull. 58(6) (2010) 782-787.

[44] A. Srinatha, J.K. Pandit, S. Singh, Ionic cross-linkined chitosan beads for extenteded release Ciprofloxacin hydrochloride: In-vitro characterization, Indian J. Pharm. Sci. 70 (2008) 16-21.

[45] S.H. Shaha, J.K. Patel, N.V. Patel, Floating multiple unit lipid granules of gatifloxacin-gelucire 39/01: formulation optimization using factorial design, Asian J. Pharm. Sci. 5(1) (2010) 35-43.

[46] J.K. Patel, M.M. Patel, Stomach specific anti-*Helicobacter pylori* therapy: preparation and evaluation of amoxicillin-loaded chitosan mucoadhesive microspheres, Curr. Drug Delivery. 4 (2007) 41-50.

[47] M. Cuna, M.J. Alonso, D. Torres, Preparation and in-vivo evaluation of mucoadhesive microparticles containing amoxicillin-resin complexes for drug delivery to the gastric mucosa, Eur. J. Pharm. Biopharm. 51 (2001) 199-205.

[48] N. Nagahara, Y. Akiyama, M. Nakao, M. Tada, M. Kitano, Y. Ogawa, Mucoadhesive microspheres containing amoxicillin for clearance of *Helicobacter pylori.* Antimicrob. Agents Chemother. 42 (1998) 2492-2494.

[49] D. Karthikeyan, M. Karthikeyan, C. Ramasamy, Effect of different viscosity grades of HPMC on drug release profile, J. Pharm. Res. 1 (2008) 23-28.

[50] M.K. Deepaa, M. Karthikeyanb, Cefpodoxime proxetil floating microspheres: formulation and in-vitro evaluation, Iran. J. Pharm. Sci. 5(2) (2009) 69-72.

[51] S. Sarojini, A.P. Kumar, D. Pradeep, R. Manavalan, B. Jayanthi, Formulation and evaluation of albumin–chitosan floating microsphere containing clarithromycin and estimation by spectrophotometric method, Res. J. Pharm., Biol. Chem. Sci. 1(2) (2010) 207-214.

[52] N. Venkateswaramurthy, R. Sambathkumar, P. Perumal, Design and evaluation of controlled release mucoadhesive microspheres of amoxicillin for anti *Helicobacter pylori* therapy, Asian J. Pharm. 5 (2011) 238-245.

[53] S.K. Sahoo, S. Mohapatra, S.K. Dhal, B.C. Behera, B.B. Barik, Formulation of floating microspheres of ciprofloxacin hydrochloride by crosslinking technique, The Indian Pharmacist. 6(58) (2007) 65-68.

[54] M. Moogooee, H. Ramezanzadeh, S. Jasoori, Y. Omidi, S. Davaran, Synthesis and in-vitro studies of cross-linked hydrogel nanoparticles containing Amoxicillin, J. Pharm. Sci. 100(3) (2011) 1057-1066.

[55] P.S. Rajinikanth, B. Mishra, Floating in situ gelling system for stomach site-specific delivery of clarithromycin to eradicate *H. pylori,* J. Controlled Release. 125 (2008) 33-41.

[56] P.S. Rajinikanth, J. Balasubramaniam, B. Mishra, Development and evaluation of a novel floating in situ gelling system of amoxicillin for eradication of *Helicobacter pylori,* Int. J. Pharm. 335 (2007) 114-122.

Chapter II

AIM, BACKGROUND CONCEPT AND OBJECTIVES

2.1. Aim

To formulate and evaluate sunflower oil entrapped chitosan coated polymeric gel beads for stomach specific delivery of amoxicillin trihydrate for the effective treatment of *Helicobacter Pylori* (*H. pylori*) *infection.*

2.2. Background Concept

H. pylori is a small, spiral, microaerophilic, gram-negative bacteria with a 4-6 bulbous tipped unipolar-sheathed flagella at one end (Fig. 2.1), which helps it to penetrate the gastric mucosa and to colonize on the gastric antrum [1,2]. Infection with *H. pylori* is universally accepted as the main threat for chronic gastritis and gastric carcinogenesis at present, and was classified as a carcinogen by the World Health Organization(WHO) in 1994 [3].

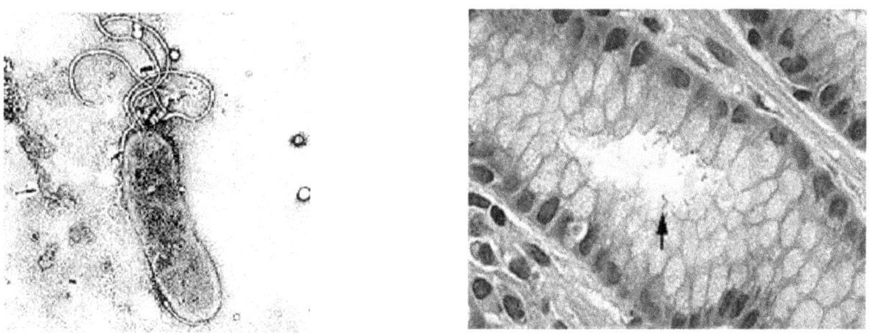

(a) **(b)**

Fig.2.1. (a) *Helicobacter pylori,* (b) Colonization of the gastric mucosa by *Helicobacter pylori* (Giemsa stain).

Estimates from the WHO in 1994 claimed that about half of the world's population was infected with *H. pylori* and although most infections are silent, a portion of the infected population will subsequently present with associated disease including chronic gastritis, peptic and duodenal ulcers (Fig. 2.2). About 550 000 new cases a year of gastric cancer-about 55% of the worldwide total-were attributed to *H. pylori,* and it was predicted that by 2020 to enter the top ten of leading causes of death worldwide [4,5].

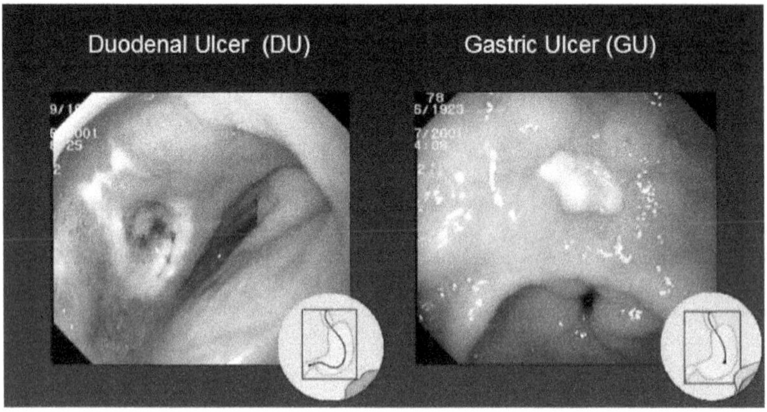

Fig.2.2. Duodenal ulcer and gastric ulcer produced by *Helicobacter pylori*

Amoxicillin (α-amino-hydroxybenzylpenicillin) is a semisynthetic, orally absorbed, broad-spectrum antibiotic. It is now widely used in a standard eradication treatment of gastric *H. pylori* infection combined with a second antibiotic and an acid-suppressing agent [6-8]. These triple therapies are proved to be effective in clinical application. However, some other reports and clinical trials indicate that the therapies cannot bring out complete eradication of *H. pylori* and suggest that the therapeutic effect needs more investigation [9, 10].

One reason for the incomplete eradication of *H. pylori* is probably due to the short residence time of antimicrobial agents in the stomach so that effective antimicrobial concentration cannot be achieved in the gastric mucous layer or epithelial cell surfaces where *H. pylori* exists [11, 12]. Because conventional drug delivery systems do not remain in the stomach for prolonged periods, they are unable to deliver the antibiotics to the site of infection in effective concentrations and in fully active forms. It is, therefore, necessary to design drug delivery systems that cannot only alleviate the shortcomings of conventional delivery vehicles but also deliver the antimicrobials to the infected cell lines (Fig. 2.3). The absorption of an antibiotic into the mucus through the mucus layer (from the gastric lumen) is believed to be more effective for *H. pylori* eradication than absorption through the basolateral membrane (from blood).

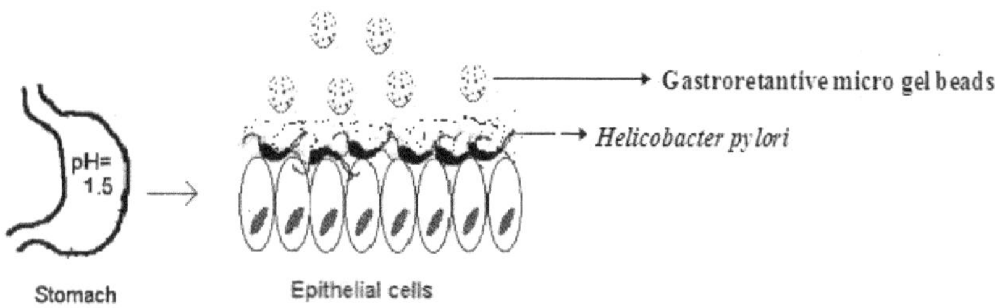

Fig.2.3. Schematics of targeted drug delivery approach for *Helicobacter pylori* eradication located within the stomach [13].

Various strategies those are currently available for the development of improved amoxicillin trihydrate loaded formulations include the formation of floating tablets, mucoadhesive tablets, mucoadhesive beads, etc., in order to retain these in the gastrointestinal tract (GIT) for an extended time to offer increased effectiveness [14-16]. Since last decade, the strategy for effective delivery of antibiotics to *H. pylori* has shifted to the use of mucoadhesive microspheres to extend the residence time in the stomach, but their drug loading capacities are poor [17,18]. On the other hand, use of biodegradable polymeric blend composites coated with a biopolymer holds a great promise to increase drug loading efficiency achieves sufficient therapeutic concentration for the treatment of gastric disease, such as peptic ulcers [19-22]. In addition, the polymeric bead formulations using vegetable oils can have a lower bulk density than gastric fluids, thereby causing the beads to float and be retained in the stomach [23, 24]. The extended retaintion of the drug can maintain a higher antibiotic concentration in the gastric region where *H. pylori* exists and thereby improve the therapeutic efficacy.

Based on this concept, we have made an attempt to develop sunflower oil entrapped buoyant gel beads of amoxicillin trihydrate using sodium algiante and hydrophilic polymer hydroxypropyl methyl cellulose(HPMC) as matrix polymers and chitosan as coating polymer. The objective of the work was to develop gel beads those will remain floated for a long time inside the stomach, delivers the drug into the gastric mucosa locally, provide a sustained action and hence increase the efficiency of the drug towards the effective treatment of *H. pylori* infection.

The polymer used, sodium alginate is an inexpensive, nontoxic product extracted from kelp. Literature reports widespread use of sodium alginate for achieving sustained release of drugs [25], targeting gastric mucosa [26] and increasing the bioavailability of drugs [27]. Additionally it also reduces interfacial tension between an oil and water phase and is efficient for preparation of emulsion. Another polymer HPMC, is a widely accepted pharmaceutical excipient, because HPMC is available in a wide range of molecular weights and the effective control of gel viscosity is easily possible. HPMC has been reported to enhance the sustained-release properties of alginate by providing a denser inner matrix [28]. Sunflower oil, the non-volatile oil compressed from sunflower (*Helianthus annuus*) seeds, also greatly aids the buoyancy of the formulation [29]. Chitosan, a polysaccharide derived from chitin by alkaline deacetylation, has been proposed as a useful coating excipient for control release of water-soluble drugs [22, 30].

2.3. Objectives

The objectives of the present work are as follows:

i. To formulate the floating beads by ionotropic gelation technique using sodium alginate and HPMC as core polymers, chitosan as coating polymer and sunflower oil as floating aid.

ii. To evaluate the formulated beads for their following physicochemical and in-vitro properties:

- Preliminary compatibility studies between amoxicillin trihydrate and polymers using FTIR spectroscopy,
- Appearance,
- Bead size and % swelling,
- Weight uniformity,
- Drug entrapment efficiency(DEE),
- Surface morphology study by Scanning Electron Microscope,
- In-vitro floating study,
- In-vitro evaluation of mucoadhesiveness,
- In-vitro drug release,
- In-vitro stability of amoxicillin trihydrate in simulated gastric fluid,
- In-vitro *H. pylori* growth inhibition study of the selected formulations,

iii. To evaluate the selected formulations for in-vivo floating.

2.4. References

[1] J.R. Warren, B. Marshall, Unidentified curved bacilli on gastric epithelium in active chronic gastritis, Lancet. 321 (1983) 1273-1275.

[2] S. Krueger, A. Roessner, D. Kuester, Murine models of *H. pylori*-induced gastritis and gastric adenocarcinoma, Pathol. Res. Pract. 207(10) (2011) 599-607.

[3] R.B. Umamaheswari, S. Jain, P.K. Tripathi, G.P. Agrawal, N.K. Jain, Floating-bioadhesive microspheres containing acetohydroxamic acid for clearance of *Helicobacter pylori,* Drug Delivery 9(4) (2002) 223-231.

[4] G.K. Tripathi, S. Singh, G. Nath, Formulation and evaluation of pH sensitive polymeric blended microgel beads of clarithromycine for the effective treatment of *Helicobacter pylori,* Der Pharmacia Sinica. 1 (3) (2010) 245-255.

[5] B.S. Dave, A.F. Amin, M.M. Patel, Gastroretentive drug delivery system of ranitidine hydrochloride: formulation and in-vitro evaluation, AAPS PharmSciTech 5(2) (2004) 77-82.

[6] I. Suleymanlar, M. Tuncer, M.T. Sezer, C. Ertugrul, M. Sarikaya, F.F. Ersoy, F. Isitan, G. Yakupoglu, G. Suleymanlar, Response to triple treatment with omeprazole, amoxicillin, and clarithromycin for *Helicobacter pylori* infections in continuous ambulatory peritoneal dialysis patients. Adv. Peritoneal Dial. 15 (1999) 79-81.

[7] N. Vakil, A. Cutler, Ten-day triple therapy with ranitidine, bismuth citrate, amoxicillin, and clarithromycin in eradicating *Helicobacter pylori,* Am J Gastroenterol. 94 (1999) 1197-1199.

[8] G.M. Buzas, E. Szekely, Eradication of *Helicobacter pylori* in peptic ulcer patients, Orv. Hetil. 140(3) (1999) 121-124.

[9] C.K. Lin, P.I. Hsu, K.H. Lai, G.H. Lo, H.H. Tseng, C.C. Lo, N.J. Peng, H.C. Chen, H.S. Jou, W.K. Huang, J.L. Chen, P.N. Hsu, One-week quadruple therapy is an effective salvage regimen

for *Helicobacter pylori* infection in patients after failure of standard triple therapy, J. Clin. Gastroenterol. 34 (2002) 547-551.

[10] E. Kawabami, S.K. Ogata, A.C. Portorreal, A.M. Magni, M.L. Pardo, F.R. Patrício, Triple therapy with clarithromycin, amoxicillin and omeprazole for *Helicobacter pylori* eradication in children and adolescents, Arq. Gastroenterol. 38 (2001) 203-206.

[11] M.P. Cooreman, P. Krausgrill, K.J. Hengels, Local gastric and serum amoxicillin concentrations after different oral application forms, Antimicrob. Agents Chemother. 37 (1993) 1506-1509.

[12] J.C. Atherton, A. Cockayne, M. Balsitis, G.E. Kirk, C.J. Hawley, R.C. Spiller, Detection of the intragastric sites at which *Helicobacter pylori* evades treatment with amoxicillin and cimetidine. Gut. 36 (1995) 670-674.

[13] P. Jansson, B. Lindberg, P.A. Sandford, Structural studies of gellan gum, an extracellular polysaccharide elaborated by *Pseudomonas elodea*, Carbohydr. Res. 124 (1983) 135–139.

[14] A.K. Hilton, P.B. Deasy, In vitro and in vivo evaluation of an oral sustained-release floating dosage form of amoxicillin trihydrate, Int. J. Pharm. 86 (1992) 79-88.

[15] M. Chun, H. Sah, H. Choi, Preparation of mucoadhesive microspheres containing antimicrobial agents for eradication of *H. pylori,* Int. J. Pharm. 297 (2005) 172-179.

[16] P.S. Rajinikanth, B. Mishra, Floating in situ gelling system for stomach site-specific delivery of clarithromycin to eradicate *H. pylori*, J. Controlled Release. 125(1) (2008) 33-41.

[17] J. Wang, Y. Tauchi, Y. Deguchi, K. Morimoto, Y. Tabata, Y. Ikada, Positively charged gelatin microspheres as gastric mucoadhesive drug delivery system for eradication of *H. pylori,* Drug Delivery 7 (2000) 237-243.

[18] Z. Liu, W. Lu, L. Qian, X. Zhang, P. Zeng, J. Pan, In vitro and in vivo studies on mucoadhesive microspheres of amoxicillin, J. Controlled Release 102 (2005) 135-144.

[19] C. Remunan-Lopez, A. Portero, M. Lemos, J.L. Vila-Jato, M.J. Nu˜nez, P. Riveiro, J.M. Lopez, M. Piso, M.J. Alonso, Chitosan microspheres for the specific delivery of amoxicillin to the gastric cavity, STP Pharma Sci. 10(1) (2000) 69-76.

[20] I. Orienti, T. Cerchiara, B. Luppi, F. Bigucci, G. Zuccari, V. Zecchi, Influence of different chitosan salts on the release of sodium diclofenac in colon-specific delivery, Int. J. Pharm. 238 (2002) 51–59.

[21] X.Z. Shu, K.J. Zhu, A novel approach to prepare tripolyphosphate/chitosan complex beads for controlled release drug delivery, Int. J. Pharm. 201 (2000) 51-58.

[22] S.C. Angadi, L.S. Manjeshwar, T.M. Aminabhavi, Novel composite blend microbeads of sodium alginate coated with chitosan for controlled release of amoxicillin, Int. J. Biol. Macromol. 51 (2012) 45-55.

[23] S.K. Dey, P.K. De, T. Goswami, A. De, A. Samanta, Formulation and in-vitro evaluation of oil entrapped floating beads of azithromycin for the effective treatment of *Helicobacter pylori,* Der Pharmacia Sinica. 5(4) (2014) 32-39.

[24] S.K. Dey, A. Samanta, K. Roy, S. Ghosh, A. Ghosh, P.K. De, Formulation and in-vitro evaluation of oil entrapped buoyant beads for stomach specific delivery of metronidazole. Int. J. Pharm. Pharm. Sci. 6(9) (2014) 407-410.

[25] A.A. Badwan, A. Abumalooh, E. Sallam, A. Abukalaf, O. Jawan, A Sustained Release Drug Delivery System Using Calcium Alginate Beads, Drug Dev. Ind. Pharm. 11 (1985) 239-256.

[26] Y. Murata, K. Kofuji, S. Kawashima, Preparation of floating alginate gel beads for drug delivery to the gastric mucosa, J. Biomater. Sci., Polym. Ed. 14 (2003) 581-588.

[27] F. Stops, J.T. Fell, J.H. Collett, L.G. Martini, H.L. Sharma, A.M. Smith, Citric acid prolongs the gastro-retention of a floating dosage form and increases bioavailability of riboflavin in the fasted state, Int. J. Pharm. 2006, 308, 14-24.

[28] P. Giunchedi, E. Gavini, M.D.L. Moretti, G. Pirisino, Evaluation of alginate compressed matrices as prolonged drug delivery systems, AAPS PharmSciTech. 1(3) (2000) 31-36.

[29] R. Bera, B. Mandal, M. Bhowmik, S.K. Dey, H. Bera, G. Nandi, L.K. Ghosh, Formulation and *In Vitro* Evaluation of Sunflower Oil Entrapped within Buoyant Beads of Furosemide, Sci. Pharm. 77 (2009) 669-678.

[30] M. Narkar, P. Sher, A. Pawar, Stomach-specific controlled release gellan beads of acid-soluble drug prepared by ionotropic gelation method, AAPS PharmSciTech. 11(1) (2010) 267-277.

Chapter III

MATERIALS

3. MATERIALS

3.1. List of General Chemicals Used

i. Hydrochloric acid (AR Grade)	: E. Merck India Ltd., Mumbai.
ii. Sodium Alginate	: LOBA Cheme Pvt. Ltd., Mumbai.
iii. Hydroxy Propyl Methyl Cellulose	: E. Merck India Ltd., Mumbai.
iv. Chitosan	: Sisco Research Lab. Pvt. Ltd., Mumbai.
v. Sunflower Oil	: Agro Tech Food Ltd., Secundrabad.
vi. Calcium chloride dihydrate	: E. Merck India Ltd., Mumbai.
vii. Glacial acetic acid	: SD Fine Chem Ltd., India.
viii. Agar	: Difco Laboratories, Detroit, MI.
ix. Horse Serum	: Invitrogen, NY.
x. Iso Vitalex	: Becton Dickinson, MD.
xi. Brain Heart Infusion	: Difco Laboratories, Detroit, MI.

3.2. List of Instruments Used

i. UV Spectrophotometer	: UV- 1700, Shimadzu, Japan.
ii. Digital Balance	: Model JL1503-C, Mettler Toledo.
iii. Hot Air Oven	: Neutron Scientific Corporation, Kolkata.
iv. Dissolution Apparatus	: USP Dissolution Apparatus, Veego, Mumbai.
v. Electric Stirrer	: RQ-121/D, Remi, India
vi. Dial Calipers	: AEROSCAPE (150 x 0.2 mm).
vii. Syringe & Needle (18 G)	: Dispovan, India.
viii. Triangular Microscope	: Magnus; Model MLX.
ix. Whatman Filter Paper	: Ashless, Circular 110 mm, Dye and Satin, India

x. Magnetic Stirrer : Model: 1 MHL, Remi.

xi. Scanning Electron Microscopy (SEM) : JSM 6100 JEOL, Tokyo, Japan.

xii. Fourier transform infrared spectroscopy : Thermo Scientific, USA, Model NICOLET iS10.

xiii. X-Ray : ESCORT, 300 M.A.

xiv. Double Gas Incubator : Heraeus, Langensebold, Germany.

3.3. Drug Profile

3.3.1. Drug Name: Amoxicillin trihydrate

3.3.2. Physicochemical Properties [1, 2]**:**

3.3.2.1. Chemical Formula: $C_{16}H_{19}N_3O_5S.3H2O$

3.3.2.2. Chemical Name: 2S,5R,6R)-6-[[(2R)-2-amino-2-(4-hydroxyphenyl)acetyl]amino]-3,3-dimethyl-7-oxo-4-thia-1-azabicyclo[3.2.0]heptane-2-carboxylic acid trihydrate.

3.3.2.3. Molecular Weight: 419.45

3.3.2.4. Chemical Structure:

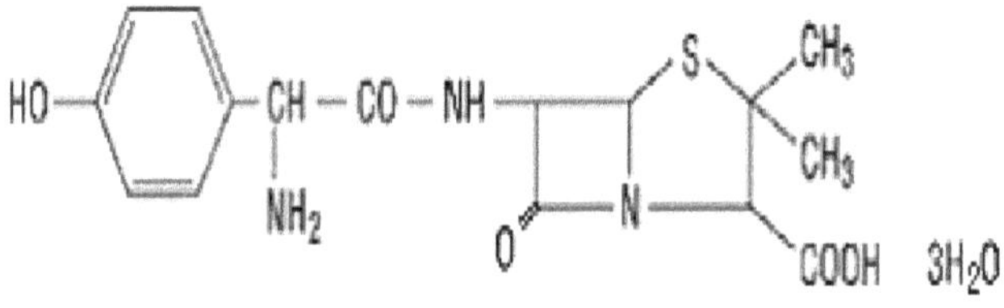

3.3.2.5. Description: White or almost white, crystalline powder. A broad-spectrum semisynthetic antibiotic similar to ampicillin except that its resistance to gastric acid permits higher serum levels with oral administration.

3.3.2.6. Solubility: Slightly soluble in water, in ethanol (95%) and in methanol; practically insoluble in chloroform, in ether and in fixed oils. It is soluble in dilute solutions of acids and of alkali hydroxides. (water solubility: 3430 mg/L)

3.3.2.7. Storage Condition: Store in tightly-closed containers in a cool place. Amoxicillin should be kept in the container it came in, tightly closed, and out of reach of children. Amoxicillin in capsules and tablets are crystalline in structure, so they should be stored at room temperature and away from excess heat and moisture (not in the bathroom). The liquid medication preferably should be kept in the refrigerator, but it may be stored at room temperature.

3.3.2.8. Melting Range: 194 °C.

3.3.2.9. Category: Antibiotic.

3.3.2.10. Heavy Metals: Not more than 20 ppm.

3.3.2.11. Category: Antibacterial.

3.3.3. Pharmacokinetics [3, 4, 5]:

3.3.3.1. Absorption: Rapidly absorbed after oral administration.

3.3.3.2. Distribution: Amoxicillin plasma protein binding is approximately 20%. The substance remains extracellular. The tissue concentrations depend on the circulation in those tissues and on the quantity of extracellular fluid. Amoxicillin diffuses adequately into the sputum, mucosa, bone tissue and aqueous humor of the eye to produce therapeutically active levels.

The concentrations in the bile are two to four times higher, or even higher than those in the blood. In the amniotic fluid and umbilical cord blood 25-30% of the mother's blood levels are attained. Amoxicillin diffuses poorly into the cerebrospinal fluid of patients with normal meninges. In inflamed meninges the concentrations are approximately 20% of those found in the blood.

3.3.3.3. Metabolism: Hepatic metabolism accounts for less than 30% of the biotransformation of most penicillins.

3.3.3.4. Elimination: Most of the amoxicillin is excreted unchanged in the urine; its excretion can be delayed by concurrent administration of probenecid. Amoxicillin is primarily eliminated via the kidneys, largely (ca. 80%) via tubular excretion, for the remainder (ca. 20%) via glomerular filtration.

Approximately 60% of an orally administered dose of amoxicillin is excreted in the urine within 6 to 8 h. Detectable serum levels are observed up to 8 h after an orally administered dose of amoxicillin.

3.3.3.5. Volume of Distribution: 0.3 L/kg.

3.3.3.6. Half life: 61.3 min.

3.3.3.7. pH: 3.5-5.5

3.3.3.8. pKa: 9.48

3.3.3.9. Plasma Protein Binding: In blood serum, amoxicillin is approximately 20% protein-bound.

3.3.3.10. Dose: The equivalent of 750 mg to 4.5 g of amoxicillin daily, in divided doses.

3.3.4. Pharmacodynamics [3-5]:

Amoxicillin is a moderate-spectrum antibiotic active against a wide range of gram-positive, and a limited range of gram-negative organisms. It is usually the drug of choice within the class because it is better absorbed, following oral administration, than other beta-lactam antibiotics.

Amoxicillin is stable in presence of gastric juices and it also produces less gastric disturbance and has the same antibacterial activity as ampicillin. It is a drug of choice in treatment of typhoid, meningitis, endocarditis, septicaemia, peritonitis and gonorrhoea. Another advantage of amoxicillin is that it penetrates equally well in to the purulent and mucoid sputum in distinction to ampicillin which does not cross the bronchial mucosa.

Amoxicillin is in the free acid form is a white crystalline powder sparingly soluble in water; It is stable in acid solution and thus can be given by mouth. It is well absorbed and produces high serum levels.

Peak serum concentrations are obtained within 60 to 90 minutes after drug administration. Animal studies demonstrated that amoxicillin is distributed evenly throughout the body tissues and is concentrated in the liver and kidneys. Small quantities enter the non infected cerebrospinal fluid. Administration of high doses results in proportionate increase in serum levels in patients with normal renal function. The drug is excreted in an active form in urine.

3.3.5. Pharmacology [3-5]:

3.3.5.1. Mechanism of Action: Amoxicillin binds to penicillin-binding protein 1A (PBP-1A) located inside the bacterial cell well. Penicillins acylate the penicillin-sensitive transpeptidase C-terminal domain by opening the lactam ring. This inactivation of the enzyme prevents the formation of a cross-link of two linear peptidoglycan strands, inhibiting the third and last stage of bacterial cell wall synthesis. Cell lysis is then mediated by bacterial cell wall autolytic enzymes such as autolysins; it is possible that amoxicillin interferes with an autolysin inhibitor.

Bactericidal; inhibit bacterial cell wall synthesis. Action is dependent on the ability of penicillins to reach and bind penicillin-binding proteins (PBPs) located on the inner membrane of the bacterial cell wall.

The more rapid bactericidal activity is linked with a different effect on the growing cells. Thus while ampicillin and some other antibiotics such as cephalexin interfare primary with septation, resulting initially in elongated filamentous forms of gram negative bacteria, amoxicillin causes rapid interference with the cell wall leading to the formation of spheroplasts and lysis.

The cell wall of bacteria is essential for the normal growth and development. Peptidoglycan is a heteropolymeric component of the cell wall that provides rigid mechanical stability by virtue of its highly cross linked lattice work structure. In gram positive organism the cell wall is 50 to 100 molecules thick, while in gram negative micro organisms it is only 1 or 2 molecules thick. The biosynthesis of peptidoglycan involves about thirty bacterial enzymes and may be considered in three stages, which are as follows:

- The first stage involves the precursor formation which takes place in cytoplasm. The product, uridinediphosphate (UDP) accumulates in the synthesis of this compound is the addition of a dipeptide. D-alanyl-D alanine.
- During reactions of the second stage, UDP acetylmuramylpentapeptide and UDP acetylglucoseamine is linked to form a long polymer. To form this species, the sugar pentapeptide is first attached by a pyrophosphate bridge to a phospholipid in the cell membrane. The second sugar is then added, followed by the addition of five glycine residue as a branch of the heteropentapeptide. The molecule is then assumed to flip across the cell membrane such that the peptidoglycan precursor faces the periplasm. The completed unit is then cleaved from the membrane bound phospholipid.
- The final stage involves the completion of the cross link. This is accomplished by a transpeptidation reaction that occurs outside the cell membrane. The transpeptidase itself is membrane bound. The terminal glycine residue of the pentaglycine bridge is linked with the fourth residue of the pentapeptide (D-alanine) releasing the fifth residue (also D-alanine). It is this last step in peptidoglycan synthesis that is inhibited by the beta lactam antibiotics.

The lysis of bacteria that usually follows their exposure to beta lactam antibiotics ultimately depend on the cell wall autolytic enzymes i.e. autolysins. The relationship between inhibition of penicillin binding proteins (PBP) activity and activation of autolysins is unclear. Some evidence suggests that exposure of bacteria to beta lactam antibiotics results in the loss of an inhibitor of the autolysins.

Beta lactam antibiotics can interfere with cell wall synthesis only in growing cells, but presumably this antibiotic can bind to the transpeptidase and related enzymes even in resting cells thus inhibiting the terminal stages of cell wall synthesis if growth is subsequently resumed.

3.3.5.2. Indication[6]: For the treatment of infections of the ear, nose, and throat, the genitourinary tract, the skin and skin structure, and the lower respiratory tract due to susceptible (only b-lactamase-negative) strains of Streptococcus spp. (α- and β-hemolytic strains only), *S. pneumoniae*, Staphylococcus spp., *H. influenzae*, *E. coli, P. mirabilis*, or *E. faecalis*. Also used for the treatment of acute uncomplicated gonorrhea (ano-genital and urethral infections) due to *N. gonorrhoeae* (males and females).

i. **Infections of the ear, nose, and throat:** Due to Streptococcus species. (α- and β-hemolytic isolates only), *Streptococcus pneumoniae*, Staphylococcus spp., or *Haemophilus influenzae*.
ii. **Infections of the genitourinary tract:** Due to *Escherichia coli, Proteus mirabilis,* or *Enterococcus faecalis*.
iii. **Infections of the skin and skin structure:** Due to Streptococcus spp. (α- and β-hemolytic isolates only), Staphylococcus spp., or *E.coli*.
iv. **Infections of the lower respiratory tract:** Due to Streptococcus spp. (α- and β-hemolytic isolates only), *S. pneumoniae*, Staphylococcus spp., or *H. influenzae*.
v. Gonorrhea, acute uncomplicated (ano-genital and urethral infections in males and females) due to *Neisseria gonorrhoeae*.
vi. *H. Pylori* eradication to reduce risk of doudenal ulcer.
vii. Triple therapy for *H. pylori* with clarithromycin and lansoprazole.

viii. Dual therapy for *H. pylori* with lansoprazole

3.3.5.3. Contraindications [6]: Contraindicated in patients with known serious hypersensitivity to amoxicillin or to other drugs in the same class or patients who have demonstrated anaphylactic reactions to beta-lactams.

3.3.5.4. Drug Interactions [6]:

i. **Probenecid:** Probenecid decreases the renal tubular secretion of amoxicillin. Probenecid may result in increased and prolonged blood levels of amoxicillin. The clinical relevance of this finding has not been evaluated.

ii. **Other Antibiotics:** Chloramphenicol, macrolides, sulfonamides, and tetracyclines may interfere with the bactericidal effects of amoxicillin. This has been demonstrated in in-vitro; however, the clinical significance of this interaction is not well documented.

iii. **Oral Contraceptives:** As with other antibiotics, amoxicillin may affect the gut flora, leading to lower estrogen reabsorption and potentially resulting in reduced efficacy of combined oral estrogen/progesterone contraceptives.

3.3.5.5. Overdose [6]: In case of overdose, discontinue of medication, symptomatic treatment and supportive measurements are required. If the overdose is very recent and there is no contraindication, an attempt for emesis or other means of removal of drug from the stomach may be performed. A prospective study of 51 pediatric patients at a poison-control center suggested that overdosages of less than 250 mg/kg of amoxicillin are not associated with significant clinical symptoms and do not require gastric emptying.

Interstitial nephritis resulting in oliguric renal failure has been reported in a small number of patients after overdosage with amoxicillin.

Crystalluria, in some cases leading to renal failure, has also been reported after amoxicillin overdosage in adult and pediatric patients. In case of overdosage, adequate fluid intake and diuresis should be maintained to reduce the risk of amoxicillin crystalluria.

Renal impairment appears to be reversible with cessation of drug administration. High blood levels may occur more readily in patients with impaired renal function because of decreased renal clearance of amoxicillin. Amoxicillin may be removed from circulation by hemodialysis.

3.4. Excipients Profile

3.4.1. Sodium Alginate [7]

3.4.1.1. Structure:

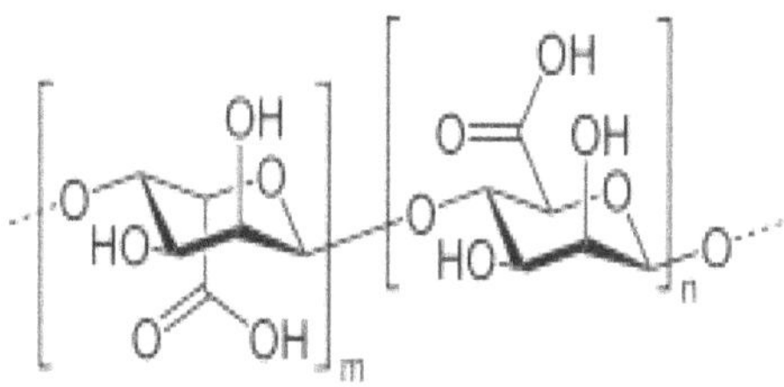

3.4.1.2. Description: A linear chain polymer extracted from seaweed composed of mannuronic acid and guluronic acid linked in the 1 to 4 positions and neutralized to form sodium salt.

3.4.1.3. Solubility: Soluble in water forming a viscous colloidal solution.

3.4.1.4. Appearance: Ivory colour, practically odorless powder.

3.4.1.5. CAS Number: 9005- 38-3

3.4.1.6. Chemical Formula: $(C_6H_7NaO_6)_n$

3.4.1.7. Formula Weight: Structural unit 198.11 (theoretical), 222 (actual average).

Macromolecule: 10,000 – 60, 0000 (typical average).

3.4.1.8. Generic Nomenclature: Algin, Sodium polymannuronate, Alginic acid and its sodium salt.

3.4.1.9. Pharmacopoeal Listing: NF, FCC (Ammonium alginate, calcium alginate, Potassium Alginate, Sodium Alginate), Codex Alimentarius.

3.4.1.10. Assay: Yeilds on the dried basis 18.00 % and not more than 21.00 % of carbon-di-oxide equivalent to not less than 90.80 % and not more than 106.00 % of sodium alginate.

3.4.1.11. Identification:

i. 0.2 gm dissolved in 20 ml of water and to 5 ml of resulting solution 1 ml of $CaCl_2$ Solutiion is added, a voluminous gelatinous precipitate is produced.

ii. To 10 ml of the solution obtained in test A 1 ml of 1M H_2SO_4 is added, a gelatinous mass is produced.

iii. 5 ml of water is added to 5 mg of sodium alginate. 1 ml of freshly prepared 1 % w/v solution of napthalene-1, 3-diol in ethanol (95 %) and 5 ml of HCl are added to it. Boiled for 3 minutes, cooled, and add 5 ml of water and shake with 15 ml of di-isopropyl ether. The upper layer exhibits a deeper bluish red color than the upper layer obtained by repeating the procedure without the substance being examined.

3.4.1.12. Purity:

i. Heavy metals: Not more than 40 ppm.

ii. Chlorides: Not more than 1.0 %.

iii. Microbial Counts: 1.0 gm must be free from *E. coli;* 10.0 gm free from salmonellae

Yeast and Moulds: Not more than 500 colonies per gram.

iv. Sulphated Ash: 30.0% - 36.0%.

v. Loss on drying: Not more than 15 % (105°, 4 h).

vi. Water insoluble materials: Not more than 2 % on the dried basis.

3.4.1.13. Uses: Thickener, suspension stabilizer.

3.4.2. Hydroxy Propyl Methyl Cellulose [8]:

3.4.2.1. Nonproprietary Names: BP/USP: Hypromellose, PhEur: Hypromellosum

3.4.2.2. Synonyms: Methyl hydroxypropyl cellulose, propylene glycol ether of methyl cellulose, methyl cellulose propylene glycol ether, methocel, HPMC.

3.4.2.3. Chemical Names: Cellulose, 2-hydroxy propyl methyl ether.

3.4.2.4. Structural Formula:

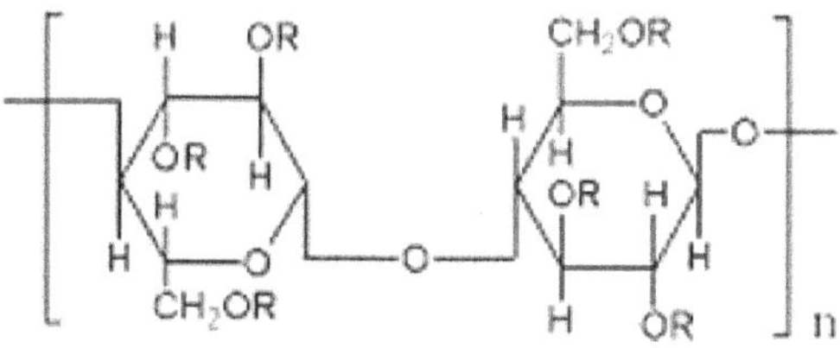

R= —H, —CH_3, or —CH_2 CH(OH)CH3

3.4.2.5. Functional Category: Suspending and /or viscosity increasing agent, tablet binder, coating agent, Viscosity increasing agent, adhesive anhydrous ointment ingredient, film former, emulsion stabilizer, rate-controlling polymer for sustain release.

3.4.2.6. Method of Manufacture: A purified form of cellulose fibers obtained from cotton linters or wood pulp, are treated with caustic (sodium hydroxide) solution. The alkali cellulose thus obtained is in turn treated with methyl chloride and propylene oxide to provide methylhydroxypropyl ethers of cellulose. The fibrous reaction product is then purified and ground to a fine, uniform powder or granules.

3.4.2.7. Description: An odorless, tasteless, white or creamy-white fibrous or granular powder.

3.4.2.8. Applications in Pharmaceutical Formulation or Technology [9, 10]: Hypromellose is widely used in oral and topical pharmaceutical formulations. In oral products, primarily used as a tablet binder, film coating material and extended release tablet matrix. Concentrations between 2 % and 5 % w/w may be used as a binder in either wet or dry granulation. Depending upon the viscosity grade, concentrations of 2-20 % w/w are used for film-forming solutions to film-coat tablets. Hypromellose is also used as a suspending and thickening agent in topical formulations, particularly ophthalmic preparations. Concentrations between 0.45-0.1 % w/w may be added as a thinking agent to vehicles for eye drops and artificial tear solutions. It is also used as an emulsifier, suspending agent, and stabilizing agent in topical gels and ointments. It is used as an adhesive in plastic bandages and wetting agent for hard contact lenses.

3.4.2.9. Typical Properties:

Acidity/ alkalinity: pH = 5.5-8.0 for a 1 % w/w aqueous solution.

Autoignition temperature: 360^{0}C

Density (bulk): 0.341 g/cm^3.

Density (tapped): 0.557 g/cm^3.

Density (true): 1.326 g/cm^3.

Melting point: Browns at 190-200^{0}C, chars at 225-230^{0}C, glass transition temperature is 170-180^{0}C.

Moisture content: Hypromellose absorb moisture from the atmosphere, the water absorbed depending upon the initial moisture content and temperature and relative humidity of the surrounding air.

Specific gravity: Approximately 1.3

3.4.2.10. Solubility: Soluble in cold water, forming a viscous colloidal solution; insoluble in alcohol, ether and chloroform, but soluble in mixtures of methyl alcohol and methylene chloride. Certain grades are soluble in aqueous acetone, mixtures of methylene chloride and isopropyl alcohol and other organic solvents.

3.4.2.11. Stability and Storage Conditions: Very stable in dry condition. Solutions are stable at pH 3-11. Aqueous solution is liable to be affected by microorganisms when used as a viscosity-increasing agent in ophthalmic solutions and anti-microbial agent. Hypromellose powder should be store in a well-closed container, cool and dry place.

3.4.2.12 Incompatibilities: Hypromellose is incompatible with some oxidizing agents. Since it is nonionic, hypromellose will not complex with metallic salts or ionic organics to form insoluble precipitates.

3.4.3. Chitosan

3.4.3.1. Description: Chitosan is a polysaccharide extracted from the shells of crustaceans, such as shrimp, crab and other sea crustaceans, including *Pandalus borealis* and cell walls of fungi.

3.4.3.2. Structure: Chitosan is also known as soluble chitin. Chitin consists mainly of unbranched chains of beta-(1→4)-2-acetamido-2-deoxy-D-glucose(=N-acetyl-dglucosamine). It is similar to cellulose, in which the C-2 hydroxyl groups are replaced by acetamido residue. Chitin is practically insoluble in water, dilute acids, and alcohol, with variation depending on product origin.

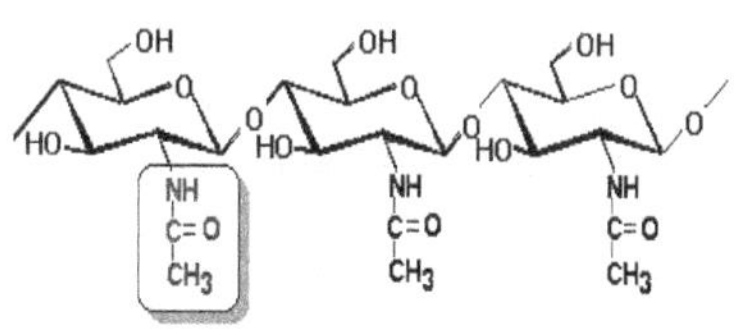

Chitin

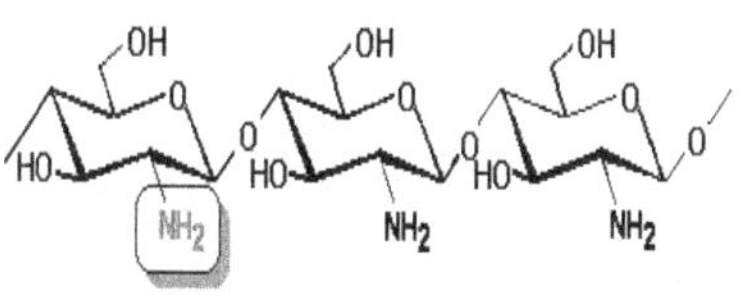

Chitosan

Chitosan, the partially deacetylated polymer of Nacetyl-D-glucosamine, is water-soluble. Structure of the chitin molecule, showing two of the N-Acetylglucosamine units that repeat to form long chains in beta-1, 4 linkages. Structure of the chitosan, composed of randomly distributed β-(1-4)-linked D-glucosamine (deacetylated unit) and N-acetyl-Dglucosamine (acetylated unit).

3.4.3.3. Chemical Name: 2-amino-2-deoxy-ß-D-glucopyranose.

3.4.3.4. Chemical Formula: $(C_6H_{11}O_4N)_n$

3.4.3.5. Preparation of Chitosan from Raw Materials: Chitosan is not a single chemical entity, but varies in composition depending on the source and method of preparation and also on physiological conditions. Chitosan could be defined as sufficiently deacetylation of chitin to form a soluble amine salts. The degree of deacetylation must be 80 to 85% or higher or the acetyl content must be less than 4-4.5% to form the soluble product. Chitosan is manufactured commercially by a chemical method. Firstly the sources such as crab or shrimp shells are washed and grinded in to powdered form and then it is deproteinized by treatment with an aqueous 3-5% solution of sodium hydroxide. After that it is neutralized and demineralized at a room temperature by treating it with aqueous 3-5% of hydrochloric solution to form a white or slightly pink precipitate of chitin. Then chitin is deacetylated by treatment with an aqueous 40-45% of sodium hydroxide solution and the precipitate is then washed with water. The insoluble part is removed by dissolving in an aqueous 2% acetic acids solution. The supernatant solution is then neutralized with an aqueous sodium hydroxide solution to obtain a purified chitosan [12].

3.4.3.6. Specification: Following table shows specification concerning chitosan [11]

Parameters	Description	Instrument
Appearance (powder or flake)	White or yellow	External shape estimation
Particle size	Less than 30 μm	Optical microscopy
Viscosity (1% solution/ 1% acid)	Less than 5 cps	Intrinsic viscosity (Capillary test)
Density	between 1.35 to 1.40 g/cm3	Densitometer
Molecular weight	50,000 to 2,00,000 Da	HPLC
pH	6.5 to 7.5	pH meter
Moisture content	More than 10 %	Gravimetric analysis
Ash value	More than 2 %	Gravimetric analysis
Matter insoluble in water	0.5 %	-
Degree of deacetylation	66 % to 99.8 %	FTIR
Heavy metal (Pb)	Less than 10 ppm	-
Heavy metal (As)	Less than 10 ppm	-
Protein content	Less than 0.3 %	Kjeldal method
Loss on drying	Less than 10 %	-
Glass transition temperature	203°C	-

3.4.3.7. Pharmaceutical Applications: Chitosan has received considerable attention as a possible pharmaceutical excipient in recent decades, due to its good biocompatibility and low toxicity properties in both conventional excipient applications as well as in novel application. Some of the general applications of chitosan in pharmaceutical fields are:

- Diluents in direct compression of tablets,
- Binder in wet granulation,
- Slow-release of drugs from tablets and granules,
- Drug carrier in micro particle systems,
- Films controlling drug release,
- Preparation of hydrogels, agent for increasing viscosity in solutions,
- Wetting agent, and improvement of dissolution of poorly soluble drug substances,
- Disintegrant,
- Bioadhesive polymer,

- Site-specific drug delivery (e.g. to the stomach or colon),
- Absorption enhancer (e.g. for nasal or oral drug delivery),
- Biodegradable polymer (implants, microparticles),
- Carrier in relation to vaccine delivery or gene therapy.

3.4.4. Sunflower Oil

3.4.4.1. Non-proprietary Name: Sunflower oil

3.4.4.2. Functional Category: Solvent and oleaginous vehicle

3.4.4.3. Origin of the Compound: Sunflower oil is the non-volatile oil compressed from sunflower (*Helianthus annuus*) seeds.

3.4.4.4. Description: Pale yellow color or yellow oily liquid, odorless.

3.4.4.5. Typical Properties:

(a) **Density**: 0.91gm/ml

(b) **Viscosity:** 0.046 Pa-S at 30.3°C

(c) **Iodine value:** 140.30

(d) **Free fatty acid content (% as oleic)** : 0.2

(e) **Peroxide value:** 0.07

3.4.4.6. Structural Formula: Sunflower oil is mainly triglycerides (fats), typically derived from the fatty acids linoleic acid (with is doubly unsaturated) and oleic acid.

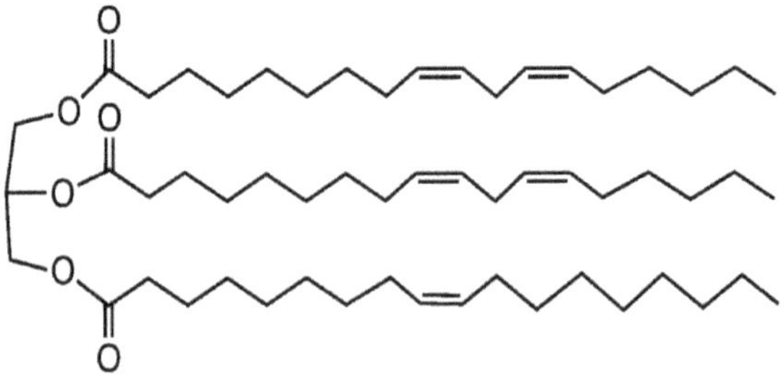

The British Pharmacopoeia lists the following profile: [13]

Palmitic acid (saturated): 5%

Stearic acid (saturated): 6%

Oleic acid (monounsaturated omega-9): 30%

Linoleic acid (polyunsaturated omega-6): 59%

3.4.4.7. Storage: Should be stored in an airtight, light resistant container protected from light and excessive heat.

3.4.4.8. Application in Pharmaceutical Formulation: Used as oily vehicle, as floating aid.

3.5. References

[1] Indian Pharmacopoeia, Fifth ed., Vol 2, The Indian Pharmacopoeia Commission, Ghaziabad, Govt. of India, Ministry of Health and Family Welfare, 2007, pp. 722-725.

[2] United States Pharmacopoeia-30 and National Formulary-25: The Official Compendia of Standards, Rockville (US): United States Pharmacopoeial Convention, 2007, pp. 1402-1407.

[3] G.E. Amidon, G.E. Peck, L.H. Block, R.C. Moreton, A. Katdare, R. Lafaver, C. Sheehan, Proposed New USP General Information Chapter, Excipient Performance (1059), Pharm. Forum. 33(6) (2007) 1311-1323.

[4] I. Legen, M. Kracun, M. Salobir, J. Kerc, The evaluation of some pharmaceutically acceptable excipients as permeation enhancers for amoxicillin, Int. J. Pharm. 308 (2006) 84-89.

[5] M.K. Goyal, S.C. Mehta, Preparation and evaluation of calcium silicate based floating microspheres of amoxicillin, J. Appl. Pharm. Sci. 1(4) (2011) 137-141.

[6] K.D. Tripathi, Essentials of Medical Pharmacology, Fifth ed., Jaypee Brothers Medical Publishers (P) Ltd, New Delhi, India, 2003, pp. 653-662.

[7] Indian Pharmacopoeia, 3rd Ed. Volume-I, 1996, pp.332-334.

[8] C.R. Raymond, L.S. Qaul, L.M. Qaul, Handbook of pharmaceutical excipients, fourth ed., Pharmaceutical Press, Royal Pharmaceutical Society of Great Britain, 2003, pp. 89-110.

[9] Z.T. Chowhan, Role of binders in moisture-induced hardness increase in compressed tablets and its effect on in-vitro disintegration and dissolution, J. Pharm. Sci. 69 (1980) 1-4.

[10] R.C. Rowe, The adhesion of film coatings to tablet surfaces- the effect of some direct compression excipients and lubricants, J. Pharm. Pharmacol. 29 (1977) 723-726.

[11] P.A. Sanford, Chitosan: Commercial uses and potential applications, in: G. Skjak-Braek, T. Anthonsen, P.A. Sanford (eds.), Chitin and chitosan: Sources, Chemistry, Biochemistry, Physical Properties and Applications, Elsevier: London, UK, 1989, pp. 51-69.

[12] J.S. Pandaya, D. Harinarayana, D. Jain, J.S. Bidkar, S. Kulthe, M.N. Kadam, An attractive biocompatible polymer for pharmaceutical application in various dosage form-chitosan, Pharmainfo. Net. 15(3) (2007).

[13] British Pharmacopoeia Commission, Ph. Eur. monograph 1371, British Pharmacopoeia, The Stationery Office, Norwich, U.K. 2005.

Chapter IV

EXPERIMENTAL WORK

Section – A

PREFORMULATION STUDY AND FORMULATION METHODOLOGY

4a.1. Standardization of Amoxicillin Trihydrate

Amoxicillin trihydrate was standardized by performing the following experimental methods:

4a.1.1. UV Scan of the Drug Sample in 0.1 N HCl:

A stock solution of amoxicillin trihydrate was prepared by accurately weighing 10 mg of the amoxicillin trihydrate in a digital balance (Model JL1503-C, Mettler Toledo) and dissolving it in 0.1 N HCl in a 100 ml volumetric flask. The volume was made up to the mark by same 0.1 N HCl solutions. 1 ml of this solution was further diluted to 100 ml with same 0.1 N HCl solution. Then the resultant solution (1 mcg/ml) was scanned by using UV Spectrophotometer (UV-1700, SHIMADZU) in the UV range of 200 to 400 nm against the same 0.1 N HCl solution as blank.

4a.1.2. Incompatibility Study Among Drug and Polymers by Fourier Transform Infrared Spectroscopy (FTIR):

Infrared spectroscopy is concerned with study of absorption of infrared radiation, which results in vibrational transitions. It is mainly used in structure elucidation to determine functional group. Every bond or portion of a molecule or functional group requires different frequency of absorption. Hence, characteristic peak is observed for every functional group or part of the molecule.

Objective:

Incompatibility is the result of mixing two or more substances which may affect the safety, efficacy and appearance of the dosage form. It is therefore of prime importance for formulation scientist to determine possible incompatibility between active ingredient(s) and excipient(s) used to make final dosage form. The main objective of this study is to find out whether there is any kind of interaction between drug and polymers present in the formulations. The incompatibility study between drug and polymer was assayed by subjecting them to infrared spectroscopy.

Methodology:

The pure drug (Amoxicillin trihydrate) and polymers (Sodium alginate, HPMC & Chitosan) were subjected to FTIR studies alone and in combination. About 3 mg of pure drug/ pure polymer/ combination of drug &polymer were grinded with 97 mg of potassium bromide in a smooth mortar to affect through mixing. The mixtures were then placed in the holder of the instrument individually and scanned individually in the mid-IR range from 400-4000cm^{-1} by using FTIR spectroscopy (Thermo Scientific, USA, Model NICOLET iS10). The detector was purged carefully by clean dry helium gas to increase the signal level and reduce moisture.

4a.2. Preparation of Calibration Curve of Amoxicillin Trihydrate in 0.1 N HCl

10 mg of the amoxicillin trihydrate was dissolved in a 100 ml volumetric flask by 0.1 N HCl. Then volume was made up to the mark by same 0.1 N HCl solutions. Different aliquots of the solution were taken in 25 ml volumetric flasks and latter volume is adjusted up to the mark by using same 0.1 N HCl solution to obtain amoxicillin trihydrate solutions of concentrations ranges from 2 mcg/ml to 40 mcg/ ml. Then each 25 ml volumetric flask gradually assayed spectrophotometrically at its maximum wave length 230.6 nm in a double beam UV and visible spectrophotometer (UV-1700, SHIMADZU) against 0.1 N HCl solution as blank. The values of absorbance were plotted against respective concentration to get the calibration curve.

4a.3. Formulation Design of Sunflower Oil Entrapped Chitosan Coated Polymeric Beads

In this design, eight (AT1 to AT8) formulations were prepared by using two levels of three experimental variables: %w/v of core polymer (Sodium alginate: HPMC=9:1), % v/v(of demineralised water) of sunflower oil and % w/v of chitosan in coating solution with the constant amount (250 mg) of amoxicillin trihydrate and water (25 ml). Formulation design datas are given in Table 4a.1.

Table 4a.1 Formulation design of sunflower oil entrapped chitosan coated polymeric beads

Batch No.	Water (ml)	Drug (mg)	Core Polymer (Na alginate: HPMC=9:1) (% w/v)	Sunflower oil (ml)	Sunflower oil (% v/v of demineralised water)	Concentration of chitosan in coating solution(% w/v)
AT1	25	250	2	1.5	6	0.25
AT2	25	250	2	1.5	6	0.75
AT3	25	250	2	2.5	10	0.25
AT4	25	250	2	2.5	10	0.75
AT5	25	250	4	1.5	6	0.25
AT6	25	250	4	1.5	6	0.75
AT7	25	250	4	2.5	10	0.25
AT8	25	250	4	2.5	10	0.75

4a.4. Preparation of Sunflower Oil Entrapped Chitosan Coated Polymeric Beads

Sunflower oil entrapped polymeric beads containing amoxicillin trihydrate were prepared by ionic gelation method. At first the aqueous slurry of sodium alginate, HPMC and amoxicillin trihydrate in demineralised water was prepared. Sunflower oil was added dropwise to the aqueous slurry with stirring at 2500 rpm by a PMDC stirrer (RQ-121/D, Remi, India) fitted with stirring shaft (6×250 mm) with pitched-blade-type propeller. The stirring was continued for 45 minutes to get a stable o/w type emulsion. The resulting drug loaded emulsions was extruded through an 18G needle into 100 ml of 5% (w/v) calcium chloride solution. After 10 min of curing time, the formed beads were washed with demineralised water and transferred to chitosan solution prepared by dissolving 0.25-0.75% w/v chitosan in 1% v/v acetic acid solution(pH adjusted to 5.0) with continuous stirring at 50 rpm on magnetic stirrer(Model 1 MHL, Remi). After 15 min, coated beads were removed, washed with demineralized and dried at 40°C for 6 h.

A total of eight formulations were prepared and the assigned formulation codes are given in table 4a.1. The flow chart of the preparation method was shown in Fig. 4a.1.

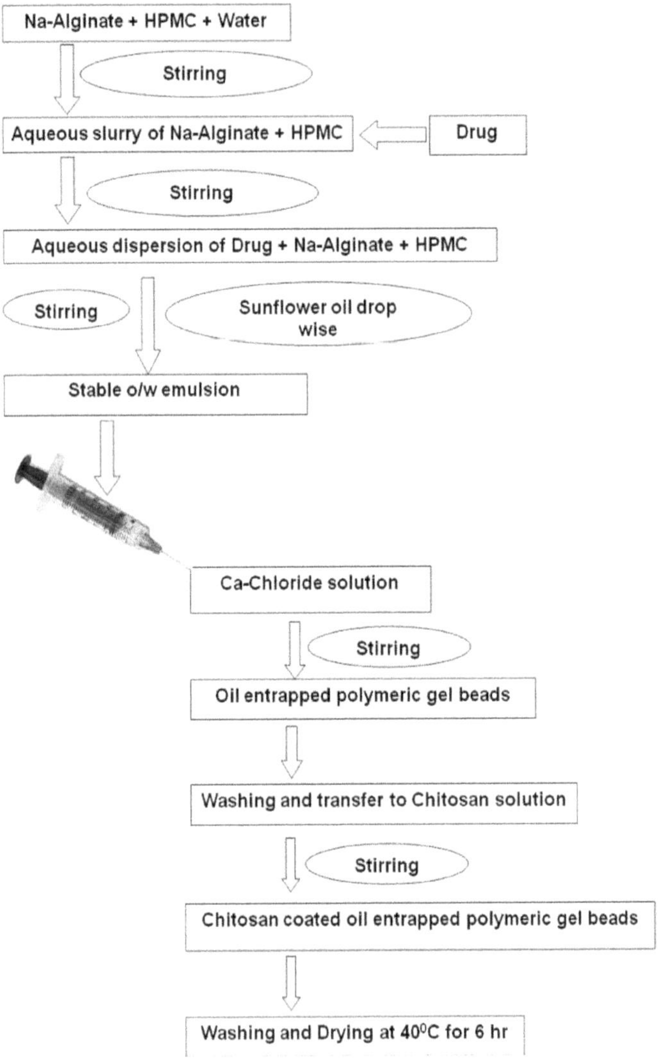

Fig.4a.1. Flow chart of the preparation of sunflower oil entrapped polymeric gel beads.

Section - B

EVALUATION

4B.1. Physicochemical Evaluation of thePrepared Beads

4b.1.1. Appearance:

Appearance of the prepared alginate beads are seen by placing them under triangular microscope (Magnus; Model MLX).

4b.1.2. Bead Size and % Swelling Measurement:

The diameter of the dried beads and wetted beads (after 8 h wetting in 0.1 N HCl were measured by Dial calipers [AEROSCAPE (150 × 0.2mm)] and the % swelling is calculated by using equation:

$$\% \text{ Swelling} = (D_2 - D_1) \times 100/D_1$$

D_1 = Diameter of the dry bead and D_2 = Diameter of the bead after swelling.

4b.1.3. Weight Uniformity Study:

To determine the weight uniformity of the various batches of beads, three sets of randomly selected 100 beads were weighed from each individual batch [1].

4b.1.4. Estimation of Drug Entrapment Efficiency:

A 100 mg portion of dried beads were placed into 100 ml of 0.1 N HCl. It was shaken over night by mechanical shaker. On the next day the resulting solution /dispersion was filtered through Whatman Filter Paper (0.45μm). The polymeric debris was washed twice with fresh buffer to extract any adhered drug. The filtrate was diluted suitably and analyzed at 230.6 nm using UV spectrophotometer (UV-1700, Shimadzu). Entrapment efficiency was calculated by using equation:

$$\text{Entrapment Efficiency} = (\text{Actual drug content} / \text{Theoretical drug content}) \times 100\ \%$$

4b.1.5. Surface Morphology Studies:

Objective:

The beads were prepared in different batches were subjected to surface study by Scanning Electron Microscope (SEM). The main objective of this study was to identify the surface characteristics and the presence of pores and the channels on the surface of the beads and also to confirm the entrapment of sunflower oil inside the bead.

Methodology:

Morphological examination of the surface and internal structure of the beads was performed by using scanning electron microscope (SEM). The samples were placed on the stubs using a carbon adhesive tape, coated with gold palladium alloy using a fine coat ion sputter (JEOL, fine coat ion sputter JFC-1100) and then surface topography was analyzed under scanning electron microscope (JSM 6100 JEOL, Tokyo, Japan) operated at an acceleration voltage of 15 kV. For examination of the internal structure of the beads, they were cut in half with a steel blade.

4b.2. In-Vitro Study

4b.2.1. Objective ofthe In-Vitro Studies:

The in-vitro studies are conducted to simulate the conditions as much as possible as in in-vivo conditions. The purpose of an in-vitro release study of a dosage form is to provide a fast, easy to perform and inexpensive method that correlates with the performance of a dosage form in human subjects. In-vitro study is also very important before in-vivo study. The in-vitro studies are very useful for many reasons, and the most obvious are only given here.

i. They are comparatively easy to perform and the effect of each parameter can be analyzed separately.

ii. The conditions of the in-vitro tests are very well defined and standardized, enabling comparison between the various results.

iii. The principle advantage is that each data set can be reduced to a simple linear equation, which replaces the tabular data.

4b.2.2. In-Vitro Floating Study:

The in-vitro buoyancy study for the beads was tested by visual observation in 0.1 N HCl. The experiment was carried out using a USP dissolution apparatus II, Veego. Twenty beads of each batch were placed into 500 ml 0.1 N HCl maintained at 37±0.5°C and 50 rpm. The time between the introduction of the beads into the medium and its buoyancy to the upper one third of the dissolution vessel (buoyancy lag time) and the time for which the formulation constantly floated on the surface of the medium (duration of buoyancy) were measured simultaneously as a part of dissolution studies [2].

4b.2.3. In-Vitro Evaluation of Mucoadhesiveness:

The sheep stomach mucosa was used for in-vitro mucoadhesion evaluation [3, 4]. The mucosa was removed and cut into pieces 2 cm long and 1 cm wide, were rinsed with 2 ml of physiological saline and fixed on glass slide. One hundred microbeads (N_0) of each were scattered uniformly on the surface of the stomach mucosa. Then, the mucosa with the microbeads was placed in a chamber maintained at 93% relative humidity and room temperature. After 20 minutes, the tissue were taken out and held at an angle 45^0. The stomach was rinsed with 0.1 N HCl for 5 minutes at a rate of 22 ml/ minutes. After 20 min beads detached from the mucosa (Ns) were observed visually and percent mucoadhesion was calculated by the following equation [5, 6].

% mucoadhesive strength= $(N_0 - Ns) \times 100/N_0$

4b.2.4. In-Vitro Drug Release Study:

For in-vitro study of the floating alginate beads USP dissolution apparatus II (Veego, Mumbai) was used. The particular amount of beads (which contained 100 mg of the drug) were placed in 500 ml of 0.1 N HCl. The stirring rate and temperature was 50 rpm and 37 ± 0.5°C respectively. Aliquots of 2 ml were withdrawn at predetermined intervals and replaced with fresh dissolution medium. Samples were suitably diluted with 0.1 N HCl up to 10 ml and assayed spectrophotometrically at λ=230.6 nm in a double beam UV and visible spectrophotometer (Shimadzu UV 1700) against 0.1 N HCl blank. The drug concentration was calculated using standard calibration curve. Finally cumulative percentage release at different time was calculated. The release data were compared with various release equations and kinetic models like zero order, first-order, Higuchi and Korsemeyer-Peppas model to investigate the drug release kinetics.

Dissolution Studies Specifications:

Dissolution Medium : 0.1 N HCl

Sample Volume : 2 ml

Replacement volume : 2 ml

Temperature : 37 ± 0.5°C

RPM : 50

Paddle Depth : 2.5cm

Dissolution medium volume: 500 ml

4b.2.5. In-Vitro Drug Release Kinetics:

For studying the release kinetics of solid, liquid or semisolid dosage forms, various mathematical models have been proposed. The in-vitro release of a drug product can be evaluated kinetically by following models:

i. Zero-Order Kinetics
ii. Noyes Whitney's rule (First Order Kinetics)[7,8]
iii. Second order kinetics
iv. Exponential release
v. Higuchi Square root equation[9-11]
vi. Hixon-Crowell Cube root equation[12]
vii. Korsmeyer-Peppas equation[13-15]
viii. Weibull function[16-18]
ix. Logarithmic-Logistics equation
x. Nernst & Brunner rule
xi. Dissolution efficiency
xii. Mean dissolution time
xiii. Other equations: Hoffenberg's equation, Davis's equation, Bamba et al equation[19]

In our study, we have used four kinetic models to evaluate in-vitro release of drug product. These models are briefly outlined below.

4b.2.5.1. Zero Order Kinetics:

Drug dissolution from pharmaceutical dosage forms that do not disintegrate and release the drug slowly (assuming the area does not change and no equilibrium conditions are obtained) can be represented by following equation: $W_0 - W_t = K.t$

Where W_0 is the initial amount of drug in the pharmaceutical dosage forms, W_t is the amount of drug in pharmaceutical dosage from at time t and K is proportionality constant. Dividing the equation by W_0 and simplifying: $f_t = K_0\, t$

Where $f_t = 1 - (W_t/W_0)$ and f_t represents the fraction of drug dissolved in time t and K_0 is the apparent dissolution rate constant or zero order rate constant. In this way, a graph of drug-dissolved fraction versus time will be linear if previously established conditions are fulfilled. This relation can be used to describe the drug dissolution of several types of modified release pharmaceutical dosage forms as in the case of some transdermal systems, as well as matrix tablets with low soluble drugs, coated forms, osmotic systems etc.

The Pharmaceutical dosage forms following this profile release the same amount of drug by unit of time and it is the ideal method of drug release in order to achieve a pharmacological prolonged action. The following relation can express this model:

$Q_t=Q_0 + K_0\, t$

Where Q_t is the amount of drug dissolved in time t, Q_0 is the initial amount of drug in the solution (most times, $Q_0 = 0$) and K_0 is zero order release constant. A plot of Q_t - Q_0 versus t gives a straight line, which passes through the origin.

4b.2.5. 2. First Order Release Kinetics:

The dissolution phenomena of a solid particle in a liquid media imply a surface action, a scan is seen by Noyes-Whitney equation:

$dq/dt = k_1 (C_s - C_t)$

Where q is the amount of drug released at time t, C_s is the solubility of the drug in the dissolution media, C_t is the concentration of the drug at time t in dissolution media and k_1 is the first order proportionality constant.

Under sink conditions, i.e., when $Ct < 0.15\, C_s$, the equation becomes:

$dq/dt = k_1 C_s$

or in integrated form, ln $q_0/q = - k_1 t$ where, q_0 is the initial amount.

A plot of log % released versus time gives a straight line with negative slope.

4b.2.5. 3. Higuchi Model:

For matrix type dosage form, the dissolution medium enters into the dosage form for the release of the drug from the matrix and the drug is diffused into the bulk solution. In such cases, Higuchi model is generally followed. The equation proposed by Higuchi is as follows:$Q = [D\,\varepsilon\,(2A - \varepsilon\,C_s)\,C_s\,t/\gamma]$

$Q = K_{HG}\,t^{0.5}$

Where Q = amount of the drug released per unit surface area of the dosage form,

D = Diffusion coefficient of the drug

ε = Porosity of the matrix

A = concentration of the drug in the matrix

C_s = Saturation solubility of the drug in the dissolution media

t = time

γ = Tortuosity of the matrix.

KHG = Higuchi release rate constant

The assumptions in deriving this equation are as follows:

(i) A pseudo-steady state is maintained during release.

(ii) A >> Cs i.e., excess solute is present.

(iii) C = 0 in solution at all times i.e., there is always sink condition.

(iv) The diffusion coefficient remains constant.

(v) No interaction between the drug and the matrix occurs.

(vi) Drug partition much smaller than these in the matrix.

For purpose of data treatment is usually reduced to $Q = KHG\,t^{0.5}$. Therefore a plot of amount of drug release from the matrix is diffusion controlled.

In this instance, one may control drug release from a homogenous matrix by varying the following parameters:

(i) Drug solubility,

(ii) Tortuosity,

(iii) Porosity,

(iv) Leaching solvent composition,

(v) Initial concentration of the drug in the matrix,

(vi) Polymer system making matrix.

The Higuchi equation postulates a diffusion controlled release mechanism.

A plot of Q Vs. $t^{½}$ yields a straight line.

4b.2.5. 4. Korsmeyer-Peppas Semi-Empirical Model

$M_t/M_\infty = k\,t^n$

Where, M_t/M_∞ is the drug fraction released at time t, k is the constant and n is the kinetic exponent of the drug release. The value of kinetic exponent indicating the mechanism of drug release process is dependent on the geometry of the systems [20]. For the case of cylindrical matrix in particular, n = 0.45 corresponds to a Fickian diffusion release (case I diffusional), 0.45 < n =0.89 to an anomalous (Non-Fickian) transport, n = 0.89 to a zero-order (case II) release kinetics, and n >0.89 to a super Case II transport.Anomalous diffusion or non-fickiandiffusion refers to combination of both diffusion and erosion controlled rate release. Case-II relaxation or super case-II transport refers to the erosion of the polymeric chain.

4b.2.6. In-Vitro Stability of Amoxicillin Trihydrate in Simulated Gastric Fluid [21]:

At first Simulated gastric fluid (SGF) without pepsin was prepared as per USP 2009. Drug loaded beads equivalent to 25 mg of amoxicillin trihydrate were placed in nine conical flasks containing100 ml of SGF, maintained at 37°C at 50 rpm in a shaking incubator. After 1, 3 and 7 h, aliquot of sample (2 ml) was withdrawn from different flasks and analyzed spectrophotometrically at 230.6 nm for drug released from beads (X_1). The remaining beads in the flasks were also recovered quantitatively, washed twice with demineralized water and air dried. The dried beads were grinded in a mortar, ultrasonicated after dispersing in 50 ml of demineralized water until complete release of the drug, and the released drug content was analyzed spectrophotometrically at 230.6 nm (X_2) to calculate percent degradation of drug using the formula:

Percent degradation = $[25-(X_1+X_2)] \times 100/25$

The similar study was carried out for plain amoxicillin trihydrate to check the percent degradation in SGF.

4b.2.7. In-Vitro *Helicobacter pylori* Growth Inhibition Study:

The *H. pylori* strain used were: 26695 (ATCC 700392) obtained from the American Type Culture Collection (ATCC, Rockville, MD). *H. pylori* were revived and cultured on brain heart infusion (BHI), agar (Difco Laboratories, Detroit, MI) supplemented with 5% horse serum (Invitrogen, NY), 0.4% IsoVitaleX (Becton Dickinson, MD), trimethoprim (5 μg/ml), vancomycin (8 μg/ml), and polymyxin B (10 μg/ml). The plates were incubated at 37°C in a microaerophilic atmosphere (5% O_2, 10% CO_2, 85% N_2) (double gas incubator; Heraeus, Langenselbold, Germany) for 3 days. Stock cultures were maintained until use at -70°C.

The growth of the bacteria was monitored by measuring the optical density (OD) of broth cultures spectrophotometrically at λ_{max} of 600 nm. The numbers of bacteria were determined in terms of optical density at λ_{max} *of* 600 nm with one optical density unit corresponding to 10^8 colony-forming units (CFU)/mL.

The plate-grown *H. pylori* strains were subcultured by inoculating to an initial optical density of 0.02 into Brucella broth containing 0.1% β-cyclodextrin at 37°C for 30 h in a microaerophilic atmosphere (5% O_2, 10% CO_2, 85% N_2).

To investigate the effect of formulations on *H. pylori* growth inhibition, 10 ml of brucella broth containing *H. pylori* were transferred into sterile test tubes. Placebo bead (without drug), plain drug and optimized batch(AT8) were taken containing amoxicillin trihydrate at a concentration of 8 μg/ml (this concentration is approximately four fold of the reported MIC50 for *H. pylori* urease) [22] and added to the tubes and all the tubes were incubated at 37°C in a microaerobic atmosphere for 24 h. The tubes containing culture were shaken at 100 rpm at 37°C in a microaerobic atmosphere condition in incubator for 24 h. Then 100μl of brucella broth of *H. pylori* containing drug and different formulations were removed at various time points (5, 10, 15 and 24 h) and OD values were checked. The percentage growth inhibition (% GI) was calculated using the following formula:

$$\% \text{ Growth inhibition} = (OD_{TP} - OD_{TS}) / OD_{TP} \times 100$$

Where, OD_{TP} = Optical density of test organism at particular interval.

OD_{TS} = Optical density of test mixture at same time interval.

4b.3. In-Vivo Floating Efficiency (X-Ray) Study of the Prepared Beads

In order to check the actual floating ability of the prepared beads on the gastric content and its usefulness in achieving to retain in stomach to increase local antimicrobial concentration, the in-vivo floating time of the formulations were determined. Batch AT8 having higher in-vitro floating was further tested for in-vivo floating. The in-vivo study was carried out by administering prepared beads to rabbits and monitoring them through a radiological method. Six healthy New Zealand breed white rabbits weighing approximately 2 to 2.5 kg were used for the study. The rabbits were fasted overnight and allowed free access to water only *ad libitum*. To make the beads opaque the incorporation of barium sulphate ($BaSO_4$) was necessary. But $BaSO_4$ has a high density (4.4777 g/cm^3) and poor floating properties. Hence, optimized floating beads were prepared by replacing a part (but not all) of the drug with X-ray grade $BaSO_4$, to improve the X-ray visibility without preventing the floatation of the beads.

X-Ray photographs were taken for the rabbits before giving the dosage form to ensure that no any radio opaque substance present inside the stomach and these photographs served as control.

Further the sunflower oil entrapped amoxicillin trihydrate loaded beads with $BaSO_4$ were administered to the rabbits using a hollow polythene tube with 3-4 ml water. About 5 to 10 ml water were further administered ensuring that the dosage form is present in the stomach and at every hour interval, 10 ml of water was administered to the rabbits throughout the study. Before taking X-ray photographs, the animals were placed/held in upright posture. At different time intervals (at 1, 4 and 6 h) for 6 h, photographs are taken by using X-Ray machine M. E. X'Ray India Pvt. Ltd., 100 M.A. to locate the position of the floating beads and to know their in-vivo floating efficiency and behavior [23, 24]. The protocol of the study was approved by Institutional Animals Ethical Committee of the Department (Ref. No. AEC/PHARM/1409/2014 Dated 14.01.2015).

4b. 5. References

[1] R. Bera, B. Mandal, M. Bhowmik, S.K. Dey, H. Bera, G. Nandi, L.K. Ghosh, Formulation and *In Vitro* Evaluation of Sunflower Oil Entrapped within Buoyant Beads of Furosemide, Sci. Pharm. 77 (2009) 669-678.

[2] B.Y. Choi, H.J. Park, S.J. Hwang, J.B. Park, Preparation of alginate beads for floating drug delivery system: effects of CO_2 gas-forming agents, Int. J. Pharm. 239 (2002) 81-91.

[3] K.V. Ranga Rao, P. Buri, A novel in situ method to test polymers and coated microparticles for bioadhesion, Int. J. Pharm. 52(3) (1989) 265-270.

[4] Y. Akiyama, N. Nagahara, T. Kashihara, S. Hirai, H. Toguchi, In vitro and in vivo evaluation of mucoadhesive microspheres prepared for the gastrointestinal tract using polyglycerol esters of fatty acids and a poly(acrylic acid) derivative, Pharm. Res. 12(3) (1995) 397-405.

[5] S. Dhawan, A.K. Singla, V.R. Sinha, Evaluation of mucoadhesive properties of chitosan microspheres prepared by different methods, AAPS PharmSciTech. 5(4) (2004)122-128.

[6] A.D. Ascentiis, J.L. deGrazia, C.N. Bowman, P. Colombo, N.A. Peppas, Mucoadhesion of poly(2-hydroxyethyl methacrylate) is improved when linear poly(ethylene oxide) chains are added to the polymer network, J. Controlled Release. 33 (1995) 197-201.

[7] J.G. Wagner, Interpretation of percent dissolved-time plots derived from in-vitro testing of conventional tablets and capsules, J. Pharm. Sci. 58 (1969) 1253-1257.

[8] M. Gibaldi, S.Feldman, Establishment of sink conditions in dissolution rate determinations: theoretical considerations and application to non-disintegrating dosage forms, J. Pharm. Sci. 56 (1967) 1238-1242.

[9] T. Higuchi, Rate of release of medicaments from ointment bases containing drugs in suspension, J. Pharm. Sci. 50 (1961) 874-875.

[10] T. Higuchi, Mechanism of sustained-action medication: theoretical analysis of rate of release of solid drugs dispersed in solid matrices, J. Pharm. Sci. 52 (1963) 1145-1149.

[11] J. Cobby, M. Mayersohn, G.C.Walker, Influence of shape factors on kinetics of drug release from matrix tablets II: Experimental, J. Pharm. Sci. 63 (1974) 732-737.

[12] A.W. Hixson, J.H.Crowell, Dependence of reaction velocity upon surface and agitation, Ind. Eng. Chem. 23(8) (1931) 923-931.

[13] R.W. Korsemeyer, R. Gurny, E. Doelker, P. Buri, N.A. Peppas, Mechanisms of solute release from porous hydrophilic polymers, Int. J. Pharm. 15 (1983) 25-35.

[14] N.A. Peppas, Analysis of Fickian and non-Fickian drug release from polymers, Pharm. ActaHelv. 60(4) (1985)110-111.

[15] R.S. Harland, A. Gazzaniga, M.E. Sangalli, P. Colombo, N.A. Peppas, Drug/polymer matrix swelling and dissolution, Pharm. Res. 5(8) (1988) 488-494.

[16] F. Langenbucher, Linearization of dissolution rate curves by the Weibull distribution, J. Pharm. Pharmacol. 24 (1972) 979-981.

[17] J.A. Goldsmith, N. Randall, S.D. Ross, On methods of expressing dissolution rate data, J. Pharm. Pharmacol. 30 (1978) 347-349.

[18] G.K. Vudathala, J.A. Rogers, Dissolution of fludrocortisone from phospholipid coprecipitates, J. Pharm. Sci. 81 (1992) 282-286.

[19] M. Bamba, F. Puisieusx, Release mechanisms in gel forming sustained release preparation, Int. J. Pharm. 2 (1979) 307-315.

[20] P.L. Ritger, N.A. Peppas, A simple equation for description of solute release. I. Fickian and non-Fickian release from non-swellable devices in the form of slabs, spheres, cylinders or discs. J. Controlled Release. 5 (1987) 23-36.

[21] S. Arora, S.Gupta, R.K. Narang, R.D. Budhiraja, Amoxicillin loaded chitosan–alginate polyelectrolyte complex nanoparticles as mucopenetrating delivery system for *H. Pylori*, Sci. Pharm. 79(3) (2011) 673–694.

[22] J.F. Tomb, O. White, A.R. Kerlavage, R.A. Clayton, G.G. Sutton, R.D. Fleischmann, K.A. Ketchum, H.P. Klenk, S. Gill, B.A. Dougherty, K. Nelson, J. Quackenbush, L. Zhou, E.F. Kirkness, S. Peterson, B. Loftus, D. Richardson, R. Dodson, H.G. Khalak, A. Glodek, K. McKenney, L.M. Fitzegerald, N. Lee, M.D. Adams, E.K. Hickey, D.E. Berg, J.D. Gocayne, T.R. Utterback, J.D. Peterson, J.M. Kelley, M.D. Cotton, J.M. Weidman, C. Fujii, C.

Bowman, L. Watthey, E. Wallin, W.S. Hayes, M. Borodovsky, P.D. Karp, H.O. Smith, C.M. Fraser, J.C. Venter, The complete genome sequence of the gastric pathogen *Helicobacter pylori*, Nature. 388(6642) (1997) 539-547.

[23] P.S. Rajinikanth, B. Mishra, Preparation and in vitro characterization of gellan based floating beads of acetohydroxamic acid for eradication of *H. pylori,* Acta Pharm. 57 (2007) 413-427.

[24] P.M. Dandag, D. Nagratna, A.P. Gadad, C.K. Pandey, V.S. Masthiholimath, Formulation and Evaluation of Itopride Hydrochloride Floating Beads for Gastroretentive Delivery, Int. J. Pharm. Sci. Nanotechnol. 6(4) (2013) 2269-2280.

Chapter V

RESULTS AND DISCUSSION

5.1. Determination of Maximum Absorbance (λ_{max}) of Amoxicillin Trihydrate

Maximum absorbance (λ_{max}) of the amoxicillin trihydrate was measured in 0.1 N HCl by using UV Spectrophotometer (UV-1700, SHIMADZU). The maximum absorbance (λ_{max}) of the amoxicillin trihydrate was found at 230.6 nm (Fig. 5.1).

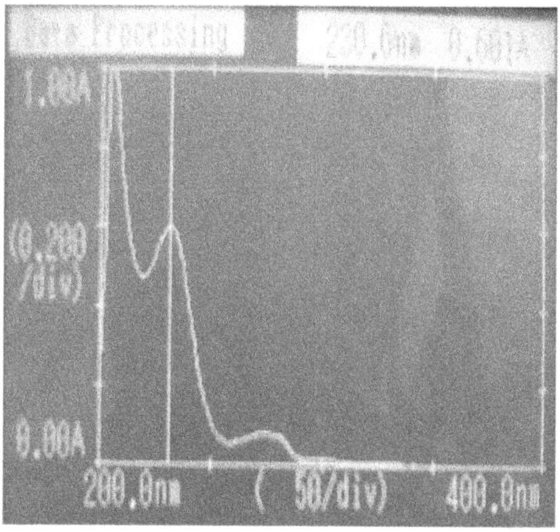

Fig. 5.1 UV Scan of amoxicillin trihydrate in 0.1 N HCl

5.2. Calibration Curve of Amoxicillin Trihydrate in 0.1 N HCl

Calibration curve of amoxicillin trihydrate was prepared spectrophotometrically in 0.1 N HCl at its maximum wave length 230.6 nm in a double beam UV and visible spectrophotometer (UV-1700, SHIMADZU) against 0.1 N HCl solution as blank. The resulted absorbances against different prepared concentrations are shown in Table 5.1. These absorbances are plotted against respective concentration to get the standard curve (Fig. 5.2.). The correlation coefficient (R^2) has been determind and found to be 0.999.

Table 5.1. Calibration curve data for amoxicillin trihydrate in 0.1 N HCl at 230.6 nm

Sl No	Concentration (mcg/ml)	Absorbance
1	2	0.059
2	4	0.099
3	6	0.149
4	8	0.198
5	12	0.302
6	16	0.41
7	20	0.517
8	24	0.617
9	28	0.82
10	40	1.018

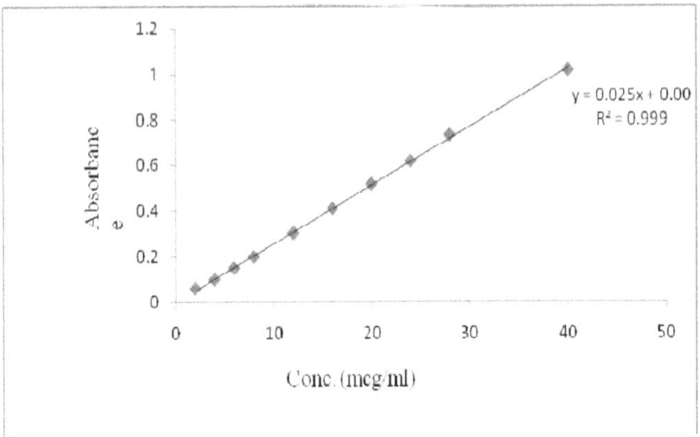

Fig. 5.2. Calibration curve of amoxicillin trihydrate in 0.1 N HCl

5.3. Fourier Transform Infrared Spectroscopy (FTIR) Study

As per the describe method FTIR was carried out for pure amoxicillin trihydrate, sodium alginate (ALG), HPMC and chitosan (CS) and physical mixture of amoxicillin trihydrate: ALG: HPMC: CS in 1:1:1 ratio. The spectrums are shown in (Fig. 5.3-5.7). The major peaks of the Amoxicillin trihydrate in its pure from and in physical mixture are tabulated in Table

5.2. From the figure it has been seen that there was no appearance or disappearance of any peak in the IR spectra. There were no major shifts in absorption bands of amoxicillin trihydrate in presence of polymers. Hence we can conclude that the drug polymers interactions were not present and amoxicillin trihydrate is fully compatible with the polymers.

Table 5.2. FTIR spectral peaks of pure amoxicillin trihydrate and combination of amoxicillin trihydrate-polymers

Spectral peaks for	Amoxicillin trihydrate	Combination of Amoxicillin trihydrate and Polymers
N-H Stretching	3465.34	3459.70
C=O (β- lactamic)	1771.88	1773.61
C=C Stretching (aromatic)	1481.63	1482.37
C-O Stretching (alcoholic)	1312.25	1312.49
C-O Stretching (phenols)	1281.78	1282.24
C-N vibration	1247.54	1249.30
C-N vibration	1177.46	1177.57
O-H Bending (alcoholic)	1144.08	1144.07
O-H Bending (alcoholic)	1120.07	1120.21
C-H Bending (aromatic)	654.43-732.40	653.84-732.78

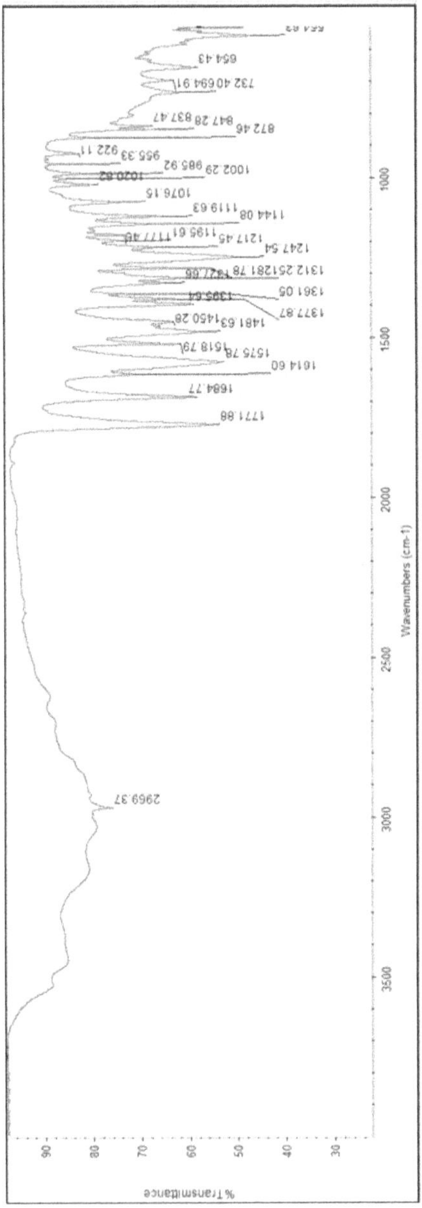

Fig. 5.3. FTIR spectrum of pure amoxicillin trihydrate

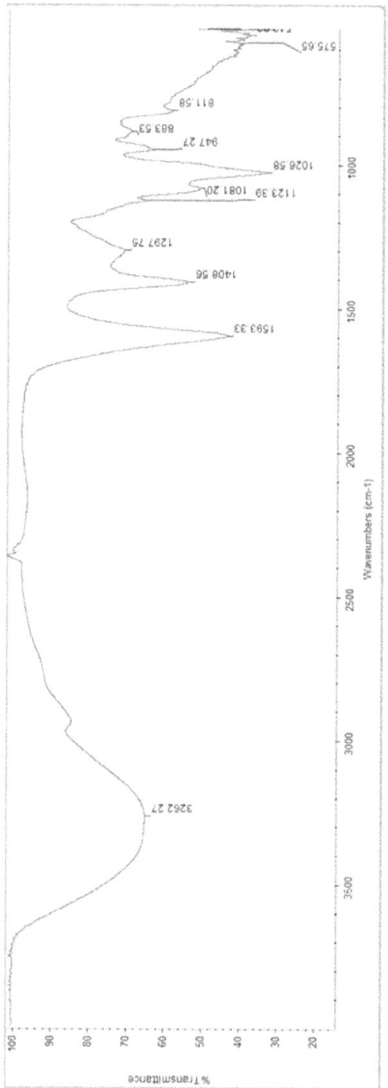

Fig. 5.4. FTIR spectrum of pure sodium alginate

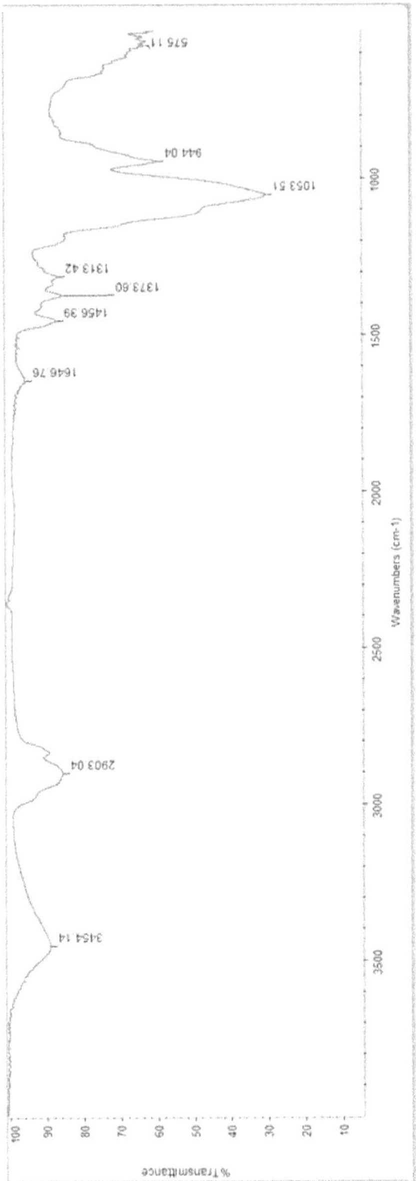

Fig. 5.5. FTIR spectrum of pure HPMC

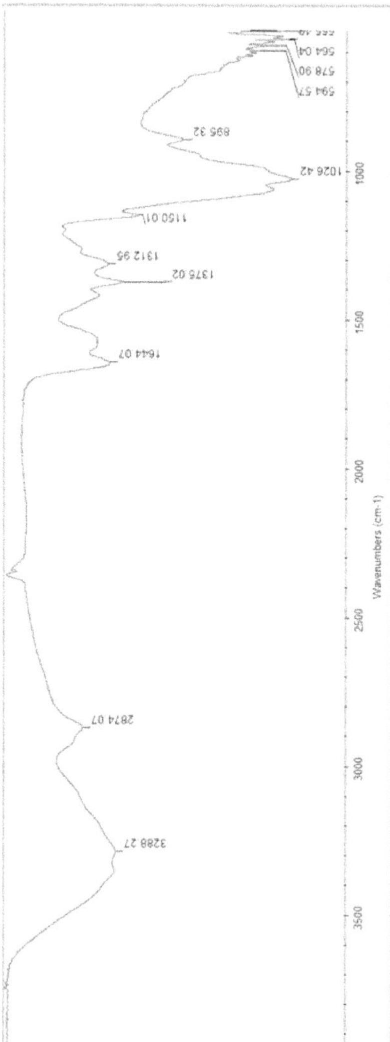

Fig. 5.6. FTIR spectrum of pure chitosan

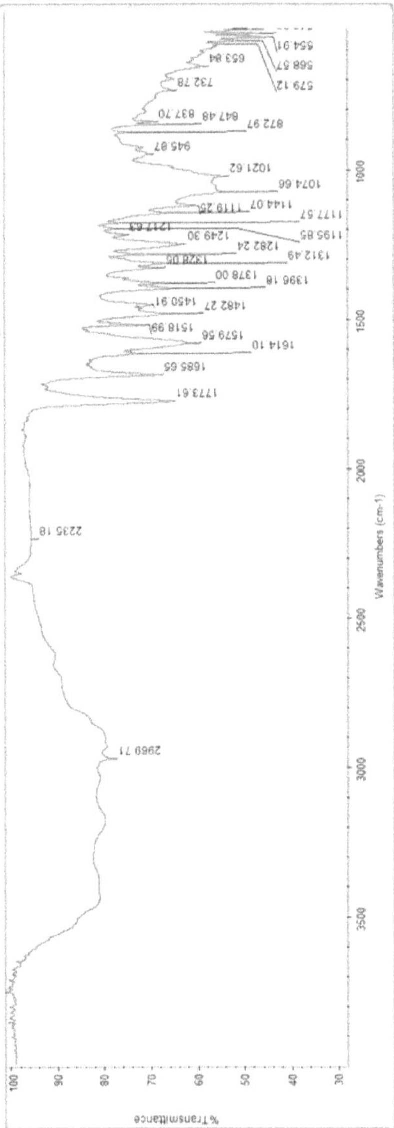

Fig. 5.7. FTIR spectrum of physical mixture of amoxicillin trihydrate, sodium alginate, HPMC, chitosan in 1:1:1:1 ratio

5.4. Formation of Gel Beads

When emulsion of sodium alginate and HPMC with sunflower oil was dropped into calcium chloride solution, spherical beads were then formed instantaneously (Fig. 5.8) due to intermolecular cross linking between the divalent calcium ions and the negatively charged carboxyl group of alginic acid, which provided a gel barrier at the surface of the formulation. Further, Chitosan coating to the formulation offered extra protection from the hars gastric environment. At slow speed of stirring, the oil get separated from the polymeric solution but high speed stirring gave the homogeneous texture of the combination because of the self-emulsifying property of sodium alginate [1]. However the emulsifying property was limited when the oil concentration was increased more than 10% v/v of demineralised water. Above this concentration, oil began to elute and leak from beads even when a homogeneous mixture was achieved.

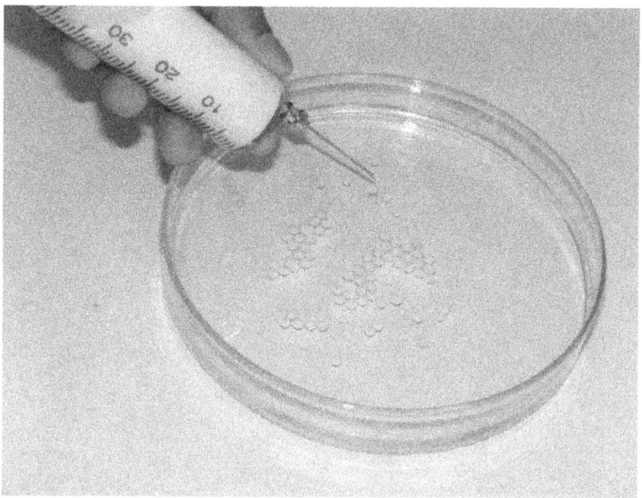

Fig. 5.8. Instantaneous formation of gel beads

5.5. Appearance

Freshly prepared beads containing sunflower oil were spherical, translucent, white and elastic (Fig. 5.9) which after drying become light brownish, smaller, dense and hard (Fig. 5.10). Brown colour is due to the original color of sunflower oil.

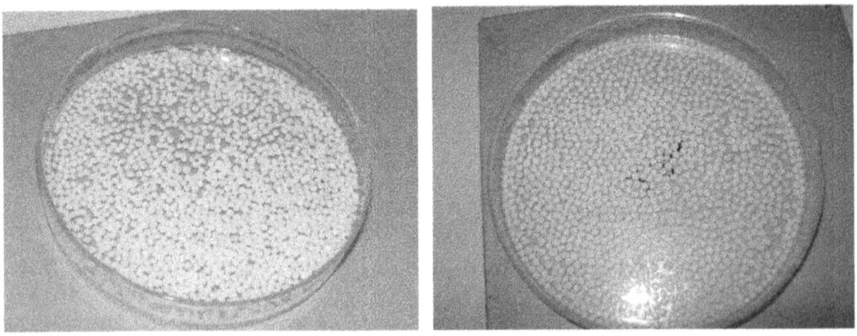

Fig. 5.9. Photographs of freshly prepared beads

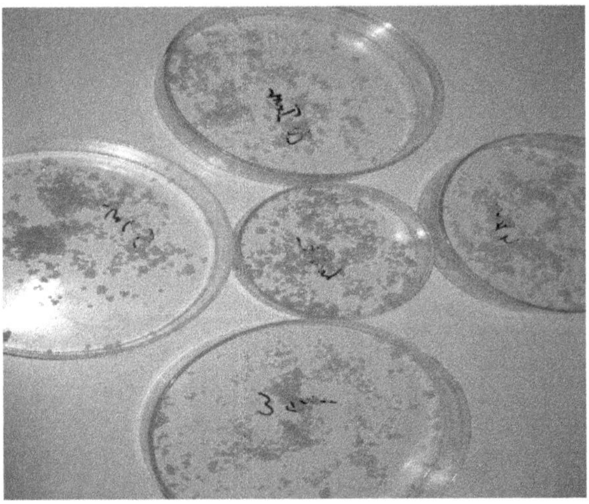

Fig. 5.10. Photograph of dried beads

5.6. Size and % Swelling

The average size of the dried beads ranged from 1.390± 0.070 mm to 1.660± 0.030 mm and sweelled beads from 1.760±0.030 mm to 2.350±0.040 mm considering the spherical shape of the beads (Table 5.3). It has been found that the diameter of dried beads was significantly increases as the concentration of core polymer increased. This is accounted for by the increased viscosity of the polymeric dispersion and consequent slow flow through the needle, which resulted in beads with bigger diameters. When the concentration of core polymer was higher than 4 % w/v, the solution with high viscosity could not form granulated beads because of the needle clogging. Therefore, no attempt for the high concentration of polymer was taken. Non spherical beads are also formed when the chitosan concentration increased above 0.75% w/v. This may be due to increase in the viscosity of the coating fluid such that the beads are irregularly coated. It was observed that amount of oil affected the morphology of the beads. An increase in oil concentration caused increase in size and sphericity of the beads. This might be due to the increased droplet viscosity by higher oil content; Droplets of lower viscosity were efficiently stirred, with a reduction in emulsion droplet size leading to smaller bead formation [2]. The mean diameter of chitosan-coated beads marginally increased with an increase in chitosan concentration (Table5.3). This could be attributed to formation of a thick chitosan coating over the beads due to its ionic interaction.

Swelling is one of the primary characteristics of the polymers used to prepare floating drug delivery system (FDDS). The outermost layer of the polymer hydrates, swells and a gel barrier is formed. Results of swelling studies are shown in Table 5.3 and Fig. 5.11. It was found that 0.75% w/v chitosan coated beads swell to a lesser extent than 0.25% w/v chitosan coated beads due to reduction of the macromolecular chain mobility, and the formation of more stable and rigid beads that show a lower tendency to swell. At lower chitosan concentration (0.25%w/v), increase in concentration of core polymer from 2%w/v (Batch

AT1 & AT3) to 4%w/v (Batch AT5 & AT7) resulted increased in swelling. But increase in core polymer concentration from 2%w/v (Batch AT2 & AT4) to 4%w/v (Batch AT6 & AT8) at high value of chitosan (0.75% w/v) resulted in lowering of swelling, which may be due to reversal of shrinkage of alginate at lower pH as well as erosion of chitosan coating in acidic environment[3]. Oil has also a little effect on swelling behavior. In batch AT1 & AT3, batch AT2 & AT4, batch AT5 & AT7 and batch AT6& AT8, the increased amount of oil in each pair of batches caused a slower swelling of beads. Thus the oil acted as a barrier for water absorption (Table 5.3 and Fig. 5.11).

Table 5.3. Size and % swelling of the prepared beads (n=3).

Batch No.	Diameter (D_1) of dried beads (mm) (Mean ± S.D.)	Diameter (D_2) of wetted beads (mm) (Mean ± S.D.)	% Swelling = (Mean D_1 – Mean D_2) x 100/Mean D_1
AT1	1.390± 0.070	2.010±0.060	44.604
AT2	1.430± 0.050	1.840±0.050	28.671
AT3	1.487± 0.071	1.977±0.085	32.952
AT4	1.510± 0.137	1.760±0.030	16.556
AT5	1.570± 0.053	2.350±0.040	49.681
AT6	1.603± 0.070	1.960±0.140	22.270
AT7	1.650± 0.030	2.250±0.100	36.363
AT8	1.660± 0.030	1.880±0.070	13.253

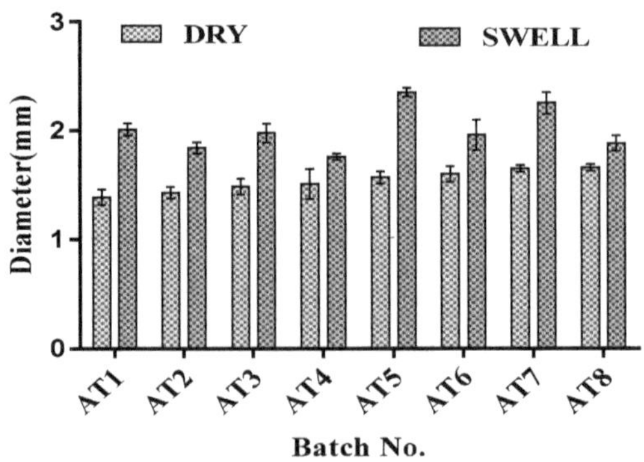

Fig. 5.11. Comparison chart of beads of different batches before and after Swelling

5.7. Weight Variation

Weight variation data (Table5.4) shows that beads are uniform in weight. Slight variation of weight is due to the bead size variation and different composition of batches. Comparision of mean weight of different batches are shown in Fig. 5.12.

Table 5.4. Weight variation data of different batches (n=3).

Batch No.	No. of beads	Weight of 100 beads (mg)			
		W_1	W_2	W_3	Mean ± S.D.
AT1	100	882.546	1002.65	848.324	911.2 ± 81.05
AT2	100	878.563	964.612	912.543	918.6 ± 43.34
AT3	100	878.564	969.111	901.145	916.3 ± 47.13
AT4	100	995.897	962.546	875.561	944.7 ± 62.13
AT5	100	908.654	999.687	860.897	923.1 ± 70.51
AT6	100	971.546	1029.21	944.987	981.9 ± 43.06
AT7	100	1017.65	870.115	965.113	951.0 ± 74.78
AT8	100	1036.46	989.561	945.129	990.4 ± 45.67

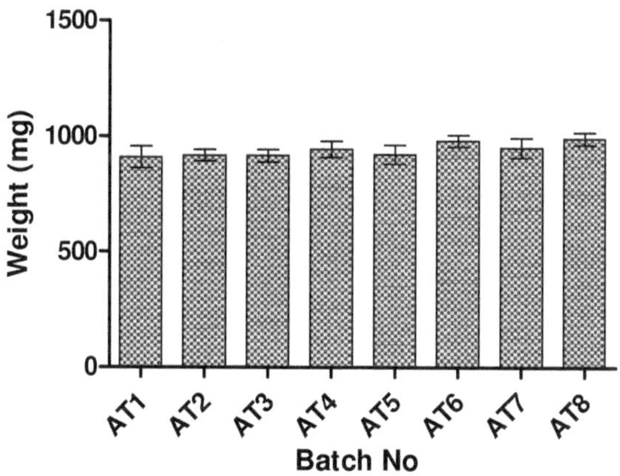

Fig. 5.12. Weight variation of different batches.

5.8. Drug Entrapment Efficiency (DEE)

Drug entrapment efficiency ranged from 55.19±4.259 % to 90.90±2.508 % depending on the composition of the eight batches of polymeric beads of amoxicillin trihydrate (Table 5.5.and Fig 5.13.). The curing time were kept to 10 minutes since drug is soluble in water. It was observed that an increase in the amount of polymer concentration also leads to increase in drug entrapment efficiency. This is because of the availability of excess of the polymer resulted in formation of larger size of beads entrapping more amount of the drug. Also the higher polymer concentration form highly dense internal structure of polymer matrix, increase bonding provides resistance to diffusion and leaching of the drug, thus increasing the entrapment efficiency. Drug entrapment efficiency was decreased with increasing oil concentration, which could be due to the replacement of the drug from the filled space of the polymer lattice. Concentration of chitosan also affects the entrapment efficiency. Again, drug entrapment efficiency increased with the increasing chitosan concentration. This phenomenon might be due to the increase in firmness of the outer barrier layer (coating) and hence reduced the diffusion rate of the drug trapped in the beads.

Table 5.5. Drug entrapment efficiency of different batches (n=3).

Batch No.	Drug content per 100 mg of the dried beads (mg)				Drug entrapment efficiency (%) Mean ± S.D.
	Theoretical (mg)	Practical (mg)			
		P_1	P_2	P_3	
AT1	2.763	1.893	2.06	1.766	55.19±4.259
AT2	4.471	3.613	3.946	3.346	65.04±5.378
AT3	2.842	2.166	2.300	2.006	60.73±4.134
AT4	4.681	4.093	4.360	3.740	69.46±5.315
AT5	2.883	3.093	3.160	2.893	84.60±3.851
AT6	4.793	5.540	5.526	5.273	90.90±2.508
AT7	2.968	2.986	3.186	2.853	81.08±4.521
AT8	5.034	5.600	5.686	5.340	88.06±2.867

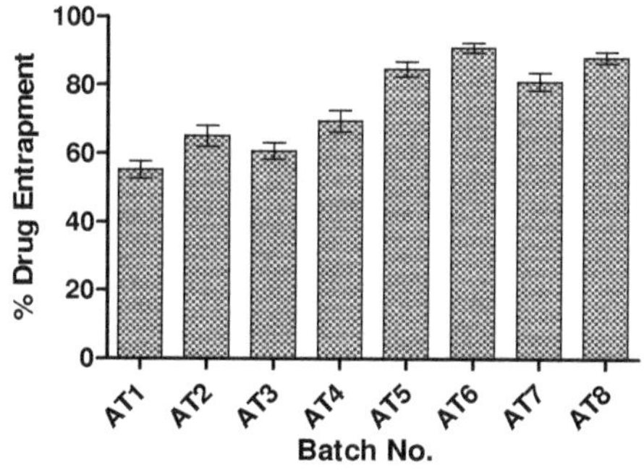

Fig. 5.13. Drug entrapment efficiency of different batches

5.9. Surface Morphology

The SEM study of the prepared beads showed almost spherical shape with few oil filled pores or channels distributed throughout (Fig. 5.14 & Fig. 5.15). The size of the pores found on the beads containing 6% v/v sunflower oil was smaller than that of the beads containing 10% v/v sunflower oil. This finding is probably due to the homogeneous dispersion of the small fraction of oil phase in polymeric solution. SEM photographs of bead cross-sections (Fig. 5.16.) revealed small pocket structures and many hollow zones with various pore diameters in all formulations. This may be attributed to the entrapment of the sunflower oil in the bead matrix. The size of these oil pockets are influenced by concentration of sunflower oil used. The large number of oil droplets in emulsion may seither tick to each other with a thin film between them, leading to flocculation, or they may coalesce into a larger droplet [4]. As a consequence, larger oil-filled pores were obtained when a greater amount (10% v/v) of sunflower oil was used to prepare the oil-entrapped beads. It has been found that when the core polymer concentration significantly increased above 4% w/v a hook with wrinkle circumference was formed (Fig. 5.17). This non-sphericity may be due to higher polymeric concentration which increases microviscosity of the polymeric dispersion and cosequent slow flow through the needle. Irregular shaped beads are also found when the chitosan concentration increased above 0.75% w/v that the viscosity of the coating fluid increased so high that uniform coating is strongly impaired.

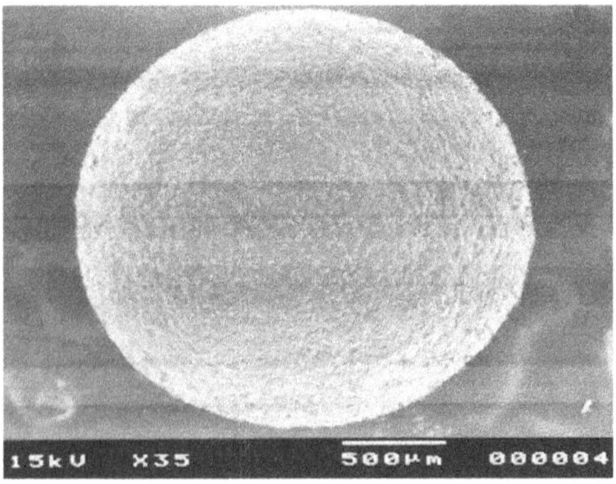

Fig. 5.14. SEM photograph of drug loaded beads showing sphericity

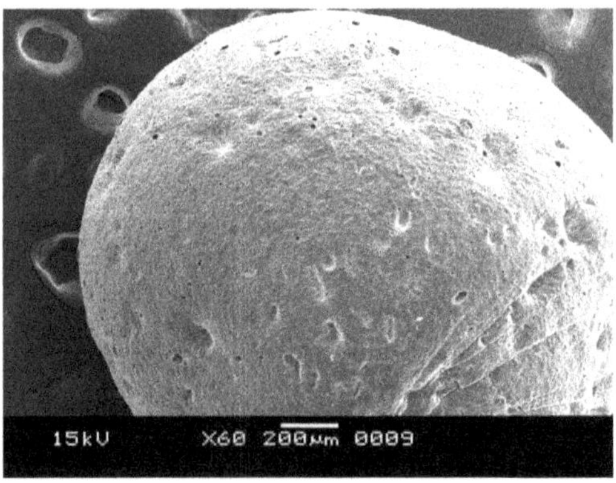

Fig. 5.15. SEM photograph of drug loaded beads showing minute channels on the surface

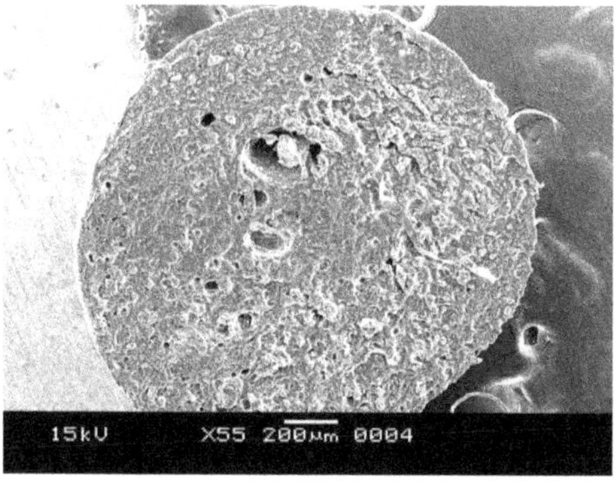

Fig. 5.16. SEM photographs of bead cross-section showing pocket structure inside

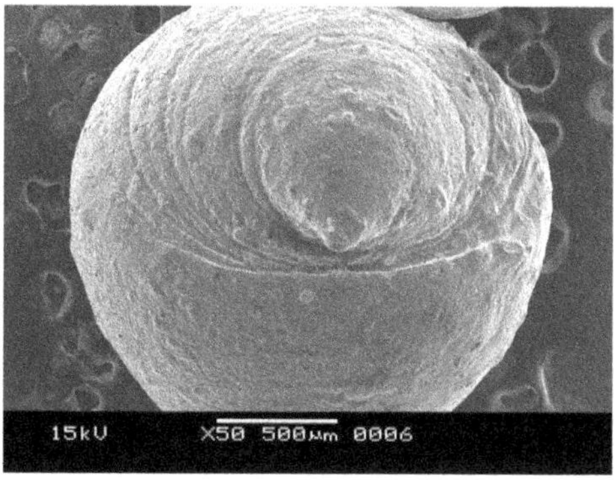

Fig. 5.17. SEM photograph of drug loaded bead showing hook formation at polymeric concentration >4%

5.10. In-Vitro Floating Study

It is evident from the result that all formulation floated within 46.33±3.215 seconds (Table5.6 & Fig. 5.18) after being placed into the acidic medium (0.1 N HCl) and remained buoyant in the medium >24 h irrespective of polymer and oil concentration. The factors contributing to the floating appeared to be the low relative densities of the sunflower oil (0.91 g mL^{-1}) as compared to that of gastric media (1.004 g mL^{-1}) and swelling. Sunflower oil serves as the dispersed phase to prepare uniform emulsion to create multiple tiny pockets in the gel matrix (observed in SEM picture) for better buoyancy. The beads with higher concentration of oil (e.g. Batch AT3, AT4, AT7 and AT8) were more flotable and took lesser lag time to float than those with lower concentrations of the oil (e.g. Batch AT1, AT2, AT5 and AT6). This may be attributed to a decrease in density of the beads with an increase in oil concentration. At the same time it was found that if the oil concentration increased above 10% v/v(results not shown) the floating time decreased which may be due to oil leakage from the formulation leading to unequal forces of released medium (0.1 N HCl) on their surfaces.

Beads coated with chitosan 0.25% w/v (Batch AT1, AT3, AT5 and AT7) showed greater lag time than with 0.75%w/v chitosan (Batch AT2, AT4, AT6 and AT8)(Table 5.6). The lower chitosan concentration may be insufficient to protect air bubbles inside the beads from the surrounding medium, leading to sinking. Batch AT8 showed minimum lag time of 25.00±5.292 sec.

Table 5.6 Lag time and floating time of different batches (n=3).

Batch No	Lag Time (Seconds)				Floating Time (Hours)
	L_1	L_2	L_3	Mean ± S.D.	
AT1	45	44	50	46.33±3.215	>24
AT2	31	45	44	40.00±7.810	>24
AT3	26	39	32	32.33±6.506	>24
AT4	26	31	20	25.67±5.508	>24
AT5	52	39	44	45.00±6.557	>24
AT6	29	30	42	33.67±7.234	>24
AT7	29	28	42	31.33±4.933	>24
AT8	21	31	23	25.00±5.292	>24

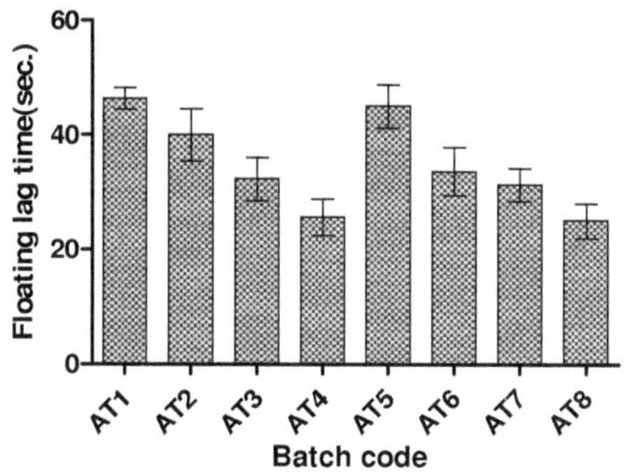

Fig. 5.18. Comparison of lag time of different batches

5.11. In-Vitro Mucoadhesiveness

All formulations have showed good mucoadhesive property (Table 5.7 & Fig. 5.19) with a mucoadhesion of 76.00 ± 2.00% to 84.67 ± 3.215%. On contact with hydrated mucous of sheep stomach tissue, microbeads swell rapidly, resulting in uncoiling of chitosan polymer chains. The cationic amino groups present on the uncoiled chitosan polymeric chains interact electrostatically with mucin glycoproteins, sialic acid and other anionic moieties present on gastric mucosa [5]. Poor swelling of alginate in acidic environment may be a reason for no further increase in mucoadhesion of microbeads at higher concentration of core polymers. Poor mucoadhesiveness at lower chitosan concentration may be due to availability of less net positive charge (amino groups) on chitosan after interaction with anionic alginate during coating process, leading to poor interaction with sialic acid and other anionic groups present on mucin [6]. There was no significant effect of the sunflower oil on the mucoadhesive property of the beads.

Table 5.7. In-vitro mucoadhesiveness of different batches (n=3).

Batch No.	Initial no. of beadsN0	Beads detached from the mucosa (Ns)			Mean % Mucoadhesiveness ± S.D.
		Ns_1	Ns_2	Ns_3	
AT1	100	25	24	22	76.33± 1.528
AT2	100	19	14	13	84.67 ± 3.215
AT3	100	18	25	24	77.67 ± 3.786
AT4	100	16	13	18	84.33 ± 2.517
AT5	100	24	26	22	76.00 ± 2.00
AT6	100	12	20	15	84.33 ± 4.041
AT7	100	24	22	20	78.00 ± 2.00
AT8	100	11	21	16	84.00 ± 5.00

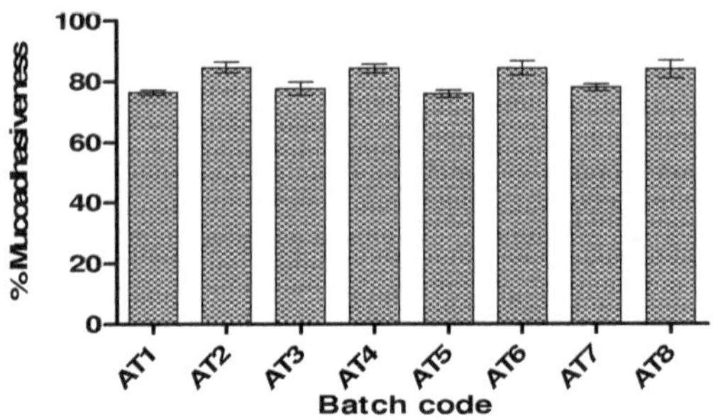

Fig. 5.19. Comparison of in-vitro mucoadhesiveness of different batches

5.12. In-Vitro Drug Release Study

Due to acid-soluble nature of amoxicillin trihydrate, it is very difficult to control its release from the prepared beads for an extended period in the acidic environment of stomach. Hence, in the present study, microgel beads were coated with chitosan to modify the drug release pattern.

Drug release pattern of the chitosan coated beads were affected by core polymer concentration, amount of sunflower oil and concentration of chitosan in coating. Cumulative

% drug release data of the all batches of the oil entrapped floating beads in 0.1 N HCl are shown in (Table 5.8.). All the batches showed a biphasic release profile as an initial small burst effect followed by a slower, gradually declining drug release phase after 1 h extending up to 7 h. This initial drug burst although small, again decreased by increased chitosan concentration. For example batch AT7 containing 0.25% w/v chitosan showed intial drug release 34.93 % at 1h where as batch AT8 containing 0.75% w/v chitosan showed intial drug release 25.10 % at 1h. This small drug burst may be due to the water-soluble nature of the drug that the drug particles were dragged on the surface of the beads during curing in aqueous surrounding medium, which are not properly protected by the thin coat of 0.25% chitosan, resulted in initial burst release but are trapped by the thick coat of 0.75% chitosan.

The results indicate that the drug release slows down with increasing core polymer concentration. It can be explained that increased of the amount of core polymer increased polymer viscosity, hence increased ionic interaction and more effectively the polymer would hold the drug with itself which resulted in decreased drug diffusion through gel matrix. Also, at low pH, the alginates do not swell, but a reversal of shrinkage takes place and the contents are not easily released [7]. Results also showed that at high concentration of core polymer, increased of chitosan concentration from 0.25% w/v to 0.75% w/v strongly decreased the drug release as found 66.97 % and 59.73 % in case of batch AT7 and AT8 respectively. This may be attributed to that thick chitosan coating not only minimizes penetration of dissolution medium but slows down the drug diffusion [8, 9]. In addition, the increased crystallinity of drug during chitosan coating may contribute for slow drug release.

Presence of oil pockets throughout the gum matrix proved by the SEM picture (Fig. 5.16.) of the cross section of the beads. After analyzing the release pattern of different batches prepared with 6% & 10% sunflower oil, it can be explained that the higher amount of sunflower oil formed a strong hydrophobic diffusional barrier retarding the drug release from the beads. It is proposed that the release of amoxicillin trihydrate in the current system is controlled by the diffusion of drug through the water-swollen polymer phase, with oil-filled droplets providing barriers, thereby increasing the tortuosity of the diffusion path.

A curve fitting method according to zero order (Fig. 5.20), first order (Fig. 5.21), Higuchi model (Fig. 5.22) for the analysis of drug release kinetics are given in Table 5.9. It has been found from the correlation coefficients of the different kinetics model that the kinetics of amoxicillin trihydrate from the system follows the Higuchi model kinetics proving that the release is by diffusion mechanism. From the results of correlation coefficients and release exponent data of different batches using the Korsemeyer–Peppas model (Fig. 5.23), it was observed that the drug release from the polymer matrix system was non fickian (anomalous transport) type ($1<n<0.5$) (Table 5.10.). Anomalous transport or non-fickian diffusion refers to combination of both diffusion and erosion controlled rate release. The initial fast release was attributed to the diffusion of the drug particles from the coating layer of the beads, while subsequent release was due to slow diffusion of the entrapped drug from the interior core of the alginate matrix

Table 5.8. Cumulative percentage amoxicillin trihydrate release of different batches at different time

Time (Hours)	AT1	AT2	AT3	AT4	AT5	AT6	AT7	AT8
0	0	0	0	0	0	0	0	0
0.5	20.4816	18.4736	20.1804	17.1684	19.8792	16.8672	18.1724	15.8632
1	40.662	35.642	39.9592	32.3288	39.658	28.0116	34.9392	25.1
2	47.7904	43.0716	44.3768	35.7424	47.0876	37.4492	42.0676	34.5376
3	53.0112	48.0916	49.5976	40.7624	51.204	42.4692	45.8828	37.9512
4	59.1356	53.8144	59.3364	51.706	60.9428	49.3968	55.4208	45.4812
5	66.8664	60.9428	63.79416	55.8224	65.40056	53.714	59.84844	47.0876
6	71.9868	66.1636	68.61336	61.0432	68.61336	58.9348	62.55924	52.8104
7	77.4084	71.5852	73.73376	68.4728	73.33216	64.0552	66.97684	59.738

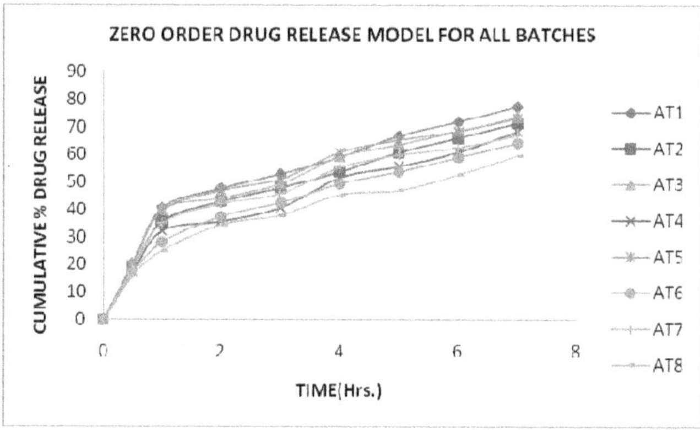

Fig. 5.20. A plot of cumulative percentage release of amoxicillin trihydrate vs. times in hour (ZERO ORDER MODEL)

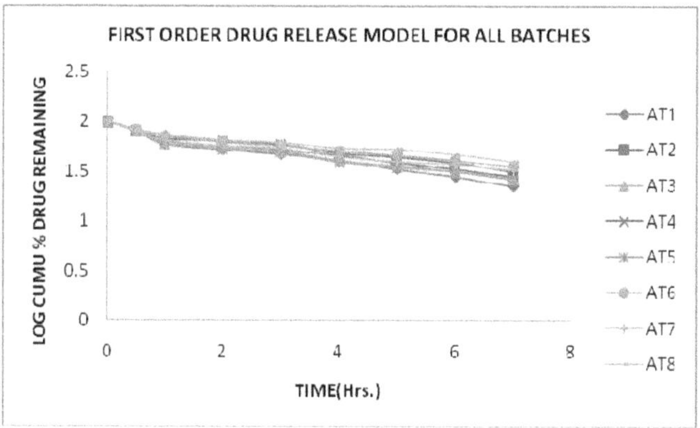

Fig. 5.21. A plot of log cumulative percentage amoxicillin trihydrate remaining to be release vs. times in hour (FIRST ORDE MODEL)

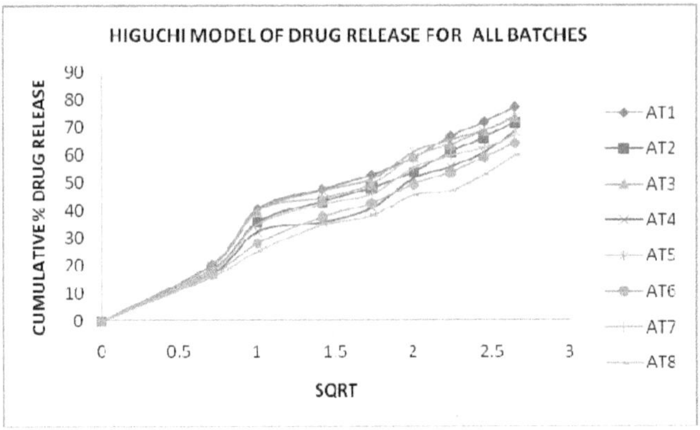

Fig. 5.22. A plot of cumulative percentage release of amoxicillin trihydrate vs. square root of time in hour (HIGUCHI MODEL)

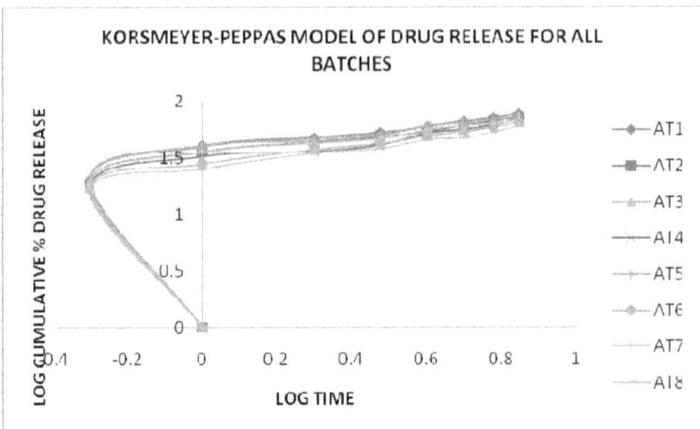

Fig. 5.23. A plot of log of cumulative percentage release of amoxicillin trihydrate vs. log time in hour (KORSEMEYER PEPPAS MODEL)

Table 5.9. Release profile of amoxicillin trihydrate from different batches showing the R^2 value in different kinetics.

Batch No.	Correlation Coefficients (R2 Value)			Model of Best Fit
	Zero Order	First Order	Higuchi	
AT1	0.856	0.962	0.976	Higuchi
AT2	0.872	0.961	0.983	Higuchi
AT3	0.852	0.955	0.974	Higuchi
AT4	0.904	0.966	0.984	Higuchi
AT5	0.836	0.946	0.971	Higuchi
AT6	0.895	0.965	0.994	Higuchi
AT7	0.850	0.941	0.977	Higuchi
AT8	0.897	0.955	0.991	Higuchi

Table 5.10. Results of correlation coefficients and release exponent data of different patches using the Korsemeyer- Peppas model

Batch No.	Correlation coefficient (R^2 value)	Release exponent (n)	Release mechanism
AT1	0.361	0.890	Non-fickian
AT2	0.376	0.889	Non-fickian
AT3	0.358	0.876	Non-fickian
AT4	0.390	0.887	Non-fickian
AT5	0.361	0.884	Non-fickian
AT6	0.397	0.887	Non-fickian
AT7	0.372	0.876	Non-fickian
AT8	0.399	0.867	Non-fickian

From the results it was found that batch AT8 had lowest in-vitro floating lag time and best control of drug release with average mucoadhesiveness and entrapment efficiency without any oil leakage and sinking (non floating) problem. Hence, batch AT8 was selected for in-vitro growth inhibition study, in-vitro stability study and for in-vivo floating study.

5.13. In-Vitro Stability of Amoxicillin Trihydrate in Simulated Gastric Fluid

The purpose of current research work was not only to control the release profile of amoxicillin trihydrate, but also to improve the stability of amoxicillin trihydrate in presence of gastric fluid. In order to examine the stability of amoxicillin trihydrate in stomach, SGF without pepsin was used as a medium for determination of relative decomposition of amoxicillin trihydrate over the period of 7 h. Decomposition of amoxicillin trihydrate in gel beads was found less than that for the pure drug (Table 5.11 and Fig. 5.24). The % degradation of amoxicillin trihydrate was decreased from 89.351 ± 2.444 % to 7.356 ± 1.201 % at 7 h by encapsulating it in microbeads (AT8) which indicated the protective efficiency of chitosan coated polymeric gel beads in gastric environment even after 7 h. This protective behaviour can be attributed to the existence of amoxicillin trihydrate in inner non-hydrated part of gel beads as in other matrix systems. Thus chitosan coated polymeric gel beads can be utilised as sustained release gastroretentive delivery system for amoxicillin trihydrate in eradication of *H. pylori* where drug formulations fail to deliver the minimum inhibitory concentration in gastric mucosa due to instability at low pH & short residence time in the stomach.

Table 5.11. Results of in-vitro stability of amoxicillin trihydrate (n=3).

Time (Hours)	% Drug degradation for plain amoxicillin trihydrate				% Drug degradation for batch AT8			
	%DD1	%DD1	%DD1	Mean±S.D.	%DD1	%DD1	%DD1	Mean±S.D.
0	2.4000	0.8000	0.0000	1.067±1.222	0.8000	0.0000	0.0000	0.267±0.462
1	18.2080	18.0960	15.7600	17.355±1.382	3.7760	5.3600	2.9600	4.032±1.220
3	40.0832	41.6816	36.0352	39.267±2.910	4.5952	6.2272	2.9792	4.601±1.624
7	91.7136	89.5056	86.8336	89.351±2.444	6.2896	7.1216	8.6576	7.356±1.201

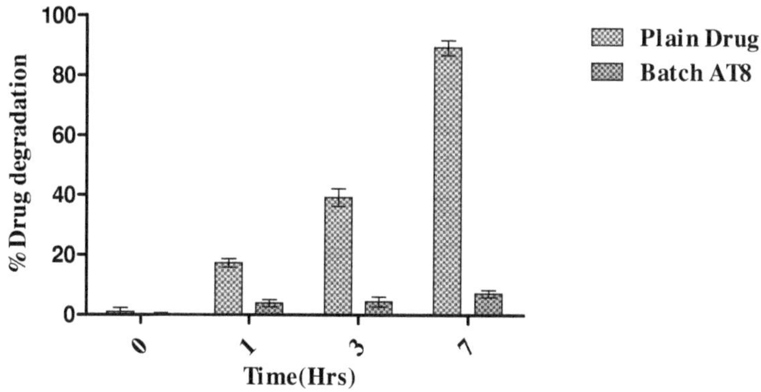

Fig. 5.24. In-vitro stability studies of amoxicillin trihydrate plain drug and batch AT8 in SGF without pepsin

5.14. In-Vitro *Helicobacter pylori* Growth Inhibition Study

Percentage growth inhibition of *H. pylori* for placebo, plain drug and chitosan coated formulation (batch AT8) was investigated at various time intervals for up to 24 h and results are shown in Table 5.12 & Fig. 5.25. The *H. pylori* culture tubes containing placebo beads (control batch) did not show any growth inhibition (maximum % GI was found to be 4.722 ± 1.248 at end of 24 h of incubation) in *H. pylori* culture (Fig. 5.25), which suggested that ingredients which are used in formulation have no anti-*H. pylori* activity. The percentage growth inhibition values injcrreased gradually with increasing incubation time. Batch AT8 showed 62.962 ± 4.625 % and 85.344 ± 5.720 % growth inhibition at the end of 5 and 10 h, respectively, where pure amoxicillin trihydrate showed comparatively more growth inhibition of 99.118 ± 1.353 % and 100% after 5 and 10 h, respectively (Table 5.12). However, the usual gastric residence of pure drug may be up to 2 h only. The drug loaded formulation (AT8) achieved complete termination of *H. pylori* infection only after 15 h of incubation.

This is because of the controlled delivery of the drug from the chitosan coated beads and the microorganisms were exposed to less of the drug where as in case of plain drug microorganisms were directly exposed to amoxicillin trihydrate. The results clearly indicate that the prepared beads of amoxicillin trihydrate have good % growth inhibition in in-vitro culture and may effectively target on the *H. pylori* surface and eradicate the *H. pylori* from the stomach. Thus, it can be expected that the prepared beads with amoxicillin trihydrate may provide the better treatment efficacy for *H. pylori* infection in-vivo.

Table 5.12. Results of in-vitro *Helicobacter pylori* growth inhibition study (n=3).

Time (Hours)	*Helicobacter pylori* growth inhibition		
	Placebo	**Amoxicillin trihydrate**	**Batch AT8**
5	0.000±0.000	99.11852±1.353	62.96296±4.625
10	1.954023±1.339	100.000±0.000	85.34483±5.720
15	2.952381±1.163	100.000±0.000	100.000±0.000
20	4.37276±1.082	100.000±0.000	100.000±0.000
24	4.722222±1.248	100.000±0.000	100.000±0.000

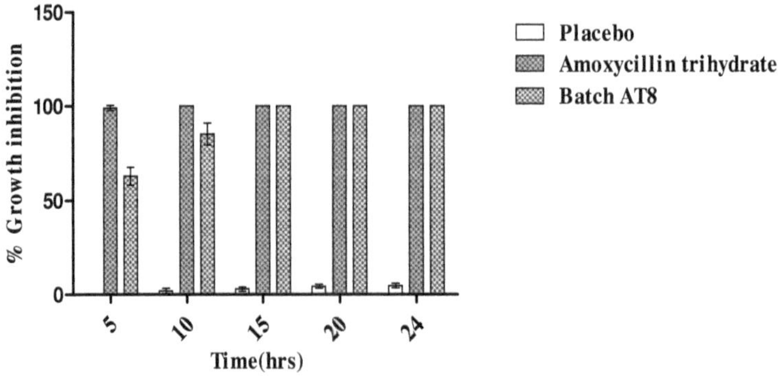

Fig. 5.25. In-vitro *Helicobacter pylori* growth inhibition of placebo beads, plain amoxicillin trihydrate and batch AT8

5.15. In-Vivo Floating Efficiency

The optimized batch AT8 had shown good in-vitro buoyancy and good release behavior and hence was finally selected for in-vivo study (i.e. X-Ray photography). After swallowing, the floating beads adopted a floating position on top of the stomach content. This might be because low relative densities of the sunflower oil and swelling. In this study, monitoring was confirmed by taking a photograph (Fig. 5.26) before giving the dosage form to ensure that no any radio opaque substace present inside the stomach and this photograph served as control. Test photographs (Fig. 5.27. to Fig. 5.29.) were taken immediately after 1, 4 and 6 h respectively. The presence of beads in stomach can be clearly noticed that, the bead remains in the stomach not being subjected to disintegration. The major limitation to the upper gastrointestinal residence time of floating dosage forms administered in the fasted state is the migrating myoelectric cycle (MMC) which cycles both through stomach and intestine every 2 to 3 h. As the results have shown that the mean gastric residence time for the developed floating beads was more than 6 h in rabbits, this means that the floating formulation withstands four of these phases without emptying. It was expected that the gastric residence of this formulations in human beings would be even longer.

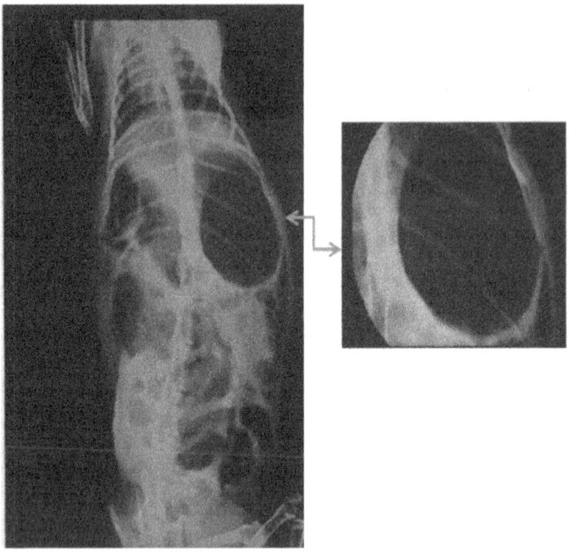

Fig. 5.26. X Ray photograph without beads

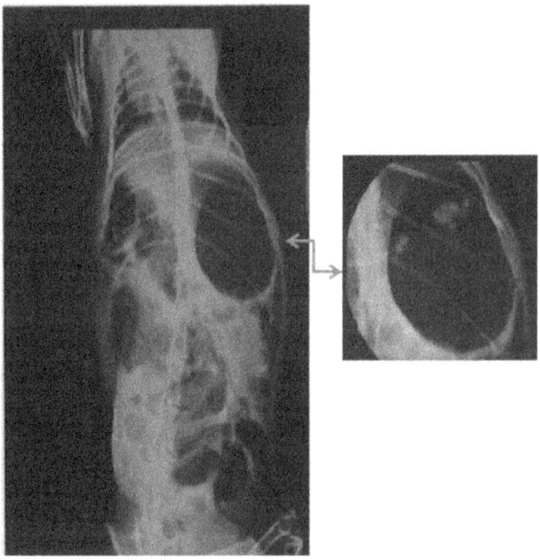

Fig. 5.27. X Ray photograph after 1 hour

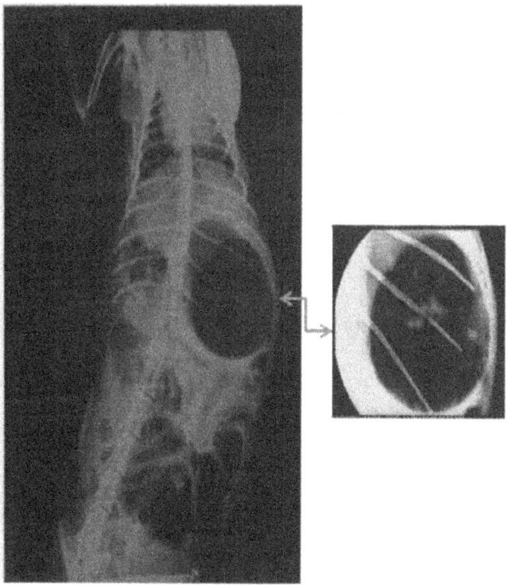

Fig. 5.28. X Ray photograph after 4 hour

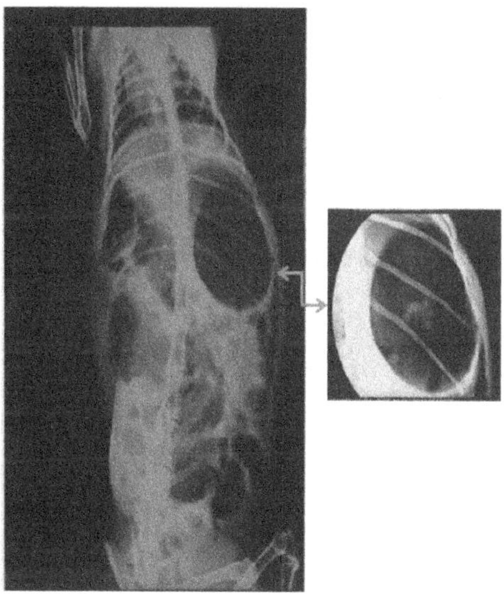

Fig. 5.29. X Ray photograph after 6 hour

5.16. References

[1] T. Yotsuyanagi, I. Yoshioka, N. Segi, K. Ikeda, Acid-induced and calcium-induced gelation of alginic acid: bead formation and pH-dependent swelling, Chem. Pharm. Bull. 39 (1991) 1072-1074.

[2] P. Sriamornsak, N. Thirawong, S. Puttipipatkhachorn, Emulsion gel beads of calcium pectinate capable of floating on the gastric fluid: effect of some additives, hardening agent or coating on release behavior of metronidazole, Eur. J. Pharm. Sci. 24 (2005) 363-373.

[3] S. Honary, M. Maleki, M. Karami, The effect of chitosan molecular weight on the properties of alginate/chitosan microparticles containing prednisolone, Trop. J. Pharm. Res. 8(1) (2009) 53-61.

[4] S.E. Friberg, R.F. Goubran, I.H. Kayali, Emulsion stability, in: K. Larsson, S.E. Friberg (Eds.), Food Emulsions, NY: Marcel Dekker, New York, 1990, pp. 1-6.

[5] M.P. Deacon, S. McGurk, C.J. Roberts, P.M. Williams, S.J. Tendler, M.C. Davies, S.S. Davis, S.E. Harding, Atomic force microscopy of gastric mucin and chitosan mucoadhesive systems, Biochem. J. 348 (2000) 557-563.

[6] C.M. Lehr, J.A. Bouwstra, E.H. Schacht, H.E. Junginger, In vitro evaluation of mucoadhesive properties of chitosan and some other natural polymers, Int. J. Pharm. 78 (1992) 43-48.

[7] S. Takka, A. Gürel, Evaluation of Chitosan/Alginate Beads Using Experimental Design: Formulation and *In Vitro* Characterization, AAPS PharmSciTech. 11 (2010) 460-466.

[8] S. Chen, M. Liu, S. Jin, B. Wang, Preparation of ionic-crosslinked chitosan-based gel beads and effect of reaction conditions on drug release behaviors, Int. J. Pharm. 349 (2008) 180-187.

[9] X.Z. Shu, K.J. Zhu, Controlled drug release properties of ionically cross-linked chitosan beads: the influence of anion structure, Int. J. Pharm. 233 (2002) 217-225.

Chapter VI
CONCLUSION

6. Conclusion

Floating drug delivery systems extend significantly the period of time over which the drugs may be released. Thus they not only prolong dosing intervals, but also increase patient compliance beyond the level of existing controlled release dosage forms. While the control of drug release profiles has been a major aim of pharmaceutical research and development in the past two decades, the control of GI transit profiles could be the focus of the next two decades and might result in the availability of new products with new therapeutic possibilities and substantial benefits for patients.

The present work demonstrated a facile approach to develop sunflower oil entrapped chitosan coated floating mucoadhesive alginate beads to increase the efficacy of amoxicillin trihydrate for eradicating *H. pylori* infection. The oil-entrapped alginate beads as core accomplished by ionotropic gelation method and were further coated with chitosan barrier. Total eight different batches are prepared varying the amount of oil (ml), polymer (mg) (Sodium alginate & HPMC) and coating agent (chitosan). The various physicochemical properties of the beads, in-vitro release of the drug, in-vitro floating time and lag time, in-vitro *H. pylori* growth inhibition, in-vitro stability of the drug and in-vivo floating time were evaluated. FTIR was also done in preformulation study to determine any kind of interactions. Surface study of the beads was also done by SEM.

These developed floating beads exhibited good mucoadhesive property (mucoadhesiveness of 76.00 ± 2.00% to 84.67 ± 3.215%), excellent drug entrapment efficiency (DEE of 55.19 ± 4.259 % to 90.90 ± 2.508 %), appreciate in-vitro buoyant ability (floating duration >24 h) with a minimum buoyant lag time (<46.33 ± 3.215 seconds), and ensure drug release beyond 7 h. Here, actually beads that were both modified with oil and coated provided the best combined buoyancy, mucoadhesion and release profile. SEM photographs revealed that the beads were spherical in shape with oil filled channels distributed throughout the surfaces. The in-vitro *H. pylori* inhibition study showed the good antimicrobial activity for formulated beads (AT8) in in-vitro *H. pylori* growth culture. Furthermore, X-ray study in rabbit stomach confirmed the gastric retention of optimized formulation (AT8) proving its efficacy as stomach-specific delivery of the drug.

The method for the preparation of floating alginate beads followed was very simple and economic. No organic solvent was used. The polymers used are biodegradable and the vegetable oil (Sunflower oil) used is an edible oil. So, this method is acceptable from Safety, Health and Environment (SHE) point of view. Therefore, the modification of calcium alginate beads with sunflower oil with further coating with chitosan can ensure the development of good floating mucoadhesive drug delivery devices for intragastric delivery of bioactive molecule in *H. pylori* eradication where drug formulations fail to deliver the minimum inhibitory concentration in gastric mucosa due to instability at low pH & short residence time in the stomach. The chitosan coated polymeric alginate beads containing sunflower oil can be given in hard gelatin capsule. It will be better to suggest administering the capsule after meal with taking one glass of water.

CPSIA information can be obtained
at www.ICGtesting.com
Printed in the USA
LVHW021426011222
734355LV00016B/982

9 781805 450726